NURSING LEADERS DRIVING HEALTH EQUITY

TACKLING SOCIAL AND STRUCTURAL DETERMINANTS

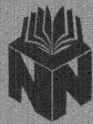

National League for Nursing

NURSING LEADERS DRIVING HEALTH EQUITY

TACKLING SOCIAL AND STRUCTURAL DETERMINANTS

Edited by:

Sandra Davis, PhD, DPM, ACNP-BC, FAANP

Andrea Lindell, PhD, RN, ANEF

. Wolters Kluwer

Philadelphia · Baltimore · New York · London
Buenos Aires · Hong Kong · Sydney · Tokyo

Vice President and Segment Leader, Health Learning, and Practice: Julie K. Stegman
Director, Nursing Education and Practice Content: Jamie Blum
Senior Development Editor: Meredith L. Brittain
Marketing Manager: Greta Swanson
Editorial Assistant: Sara Thul
Manager, Graphic Arts and Design: Steve Druding
Art Director: Jennifer Clements
Senior Production Project Manager: Catherine Ott
Manufacturing Coordinator: Margie Orzech
Prepress Vendor: Aptara, Inc.

9 8 7 6 5 4 3 2 1

Printed in the United States of America

Library of Congress Cataloging-in-Publication Data

978-1-9752-4830-7

Cataloging in Publication data available on request from publisher.

MPP0624

About the Editors

Sandra Davis, PhD, DPM, ACNP-BC, FAANP, is Deputy Chief Director for the NLN/Walden University College of Nursing Institute for Social Determinants of Health and Social Change. Prior to joining the NLN Dr. Davis was Associate Professor and Inaugural Associate Dean for Diversity, Equity, and Inclusion (DEI), at the George Washington University School of Nursing. With decades of faculty, administrative, educator, clinical practice, and leadership roles her scholarly interests include health inequities, social and structural determinants of health, structural competency, and antiracism. Dr. Davis chairs the International Council of Nurses (ICN) Education Experts Advisory Committee (ICNEE) where she brings her knowledge and experience to broadening the commitment to quality and equity in nursing education around the world. She contributed to the NLN Vision Series, A Vision for Integration of the Social Determinants of Health into Nursing Education Curricula, and sat on the National Commission to Address Racism in Nursing. Dr. Davis was Principal Investigator on a Photovoice Project: "The Social Determinants of a Heart Healthy Community" exhibited at the Smithsonian National Museum of African American History and Culture. She co-published an article in Academic Medicine entitled "Let's Talk about Racism: Building Structural Competency in Nursing." Her co-authored book *Fast Facts about Diversity, Equity, and Inclusion in Nursing: Building Competencies for an Antiracism Practice* received an AJN 3rd place 2022 book of the year award. Dr. Davis is on the editorial board for Nursing Education Perspectives and was a guest editor for the September/October 2023 special issue on Equity, Diversity, and Inclusion. Dr. Davis is a board-certified Acute Care Nurse Practitioner and Past President of the NP Association of DC. She is an AACN/Wharton Executive Leadership Fellow, a Leadership for Academic Nursing Fellow, a Fellow in AANP, and an inductee in the Temple University Distinguished Alumni Gallery of Success. Dr. Davis received a BA from Wellesley College, a BSN from Temple University, an MSN and ACNP certification from the University of Pennsylvania, a DPM from Temple University, and a PhD from Drexel University in Educational Leadership.

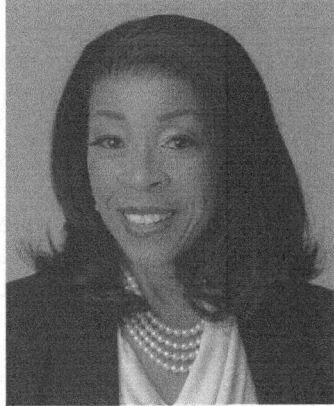

Andrea Lindell, PhD, RN, ANEF, received her PhD in Nursing, MSN at The Catholic University of America in Washington, D.C., and BSN at Villa Maria College, Erie, PA.

Dr. Lindell currently serves as Vice-Provost, Walden University. Prior to that she served as Dean of the College of Nursing at Walden University from March 2013 until 2020. She also held the title as Laureate Health Sciences Specialist from the Health Sciences Laureate International Universities for advancing the education of health professions and helping other network institutions in achieving excellence in the field of Health Sciences. Dr. Lindell also held the position of Dean and Professor, College of Nursing University of Cincinnati since 1990 until 2011 where she also held the position of Associate Senior Vice President for Academic Health Affairs in the Medical Center. Dr. Lindell also developed and supervised international collaborative academic program partnerships with Yonsi University, Seoul, Korea; Pam American University, Mexico City, Mexico; Kyoto Hospital, Kyoto, Japan; and others. Dr. Lindell was the co-founder and interim Dean of the College of Health Sciences, University of Cincinnati for 9 years. Dr. Lindell held national leadership positions as Treasurer then President of the American Association of Colleges of Nursing (AACN), University Representative and Treasurer on the Council on Accreditation of Anesthesia Educational Programs, Midwest Alliance in Nursing (MAIN) and is the current Board of Trustees member on two single-degree granting College of Nursing institutions. She served on numerous board and committee positions at the local, state, and national levels. She held director positions on two corporate boards. Currently she holds the director position on one corporate board. Dr. Lindell has authored numerous publications in referred journals and book chapters, served as journal reviewer, has given presentations nationally and internationally, and was keynote speaker at several university commencements. Dr. Lindell has served in roles as accreditation on-site reviewer and served as lead reviewer and consultant on the King Hussein Excellence in Education project for the assessment and evaluation of all nursing programs in Jordan. She is a national/international consultant in the areas of program development, curriculum design and implementation, program evaluation strategies, and accreditation readiness. Dr. Lindell has received numerous awards, such as Outstanding Leadership in Nursing, Outstanding Alumni, American Association of Colleges of Nursing National Sister Bernadette Armiger Award for Outstanding Leadership in Nursing Education (2010), and Women Worth Watching in 2015 Award by the Journal of Diversity.

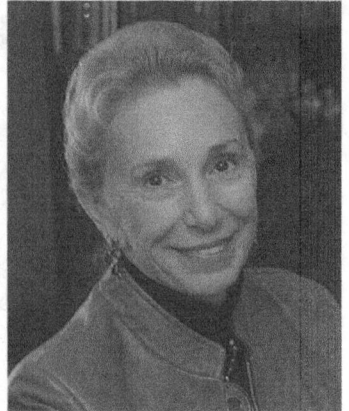

About the Contributors

Aimee Ferraro, PhD, MPH, is an epidemiologist and senior faculty at Walden University, where she has taught and developed courses in the Public Health programs for 15 years. She has extensive experience conducting mixed methods research in diverse public health settings and addressing the needs of vulnerable populations. Since completing a CDC/CSTE Applied Epidemiology Fellowship with the Pennsylvania Department of Health, her work has focused on social determinants of health and infectious diseases such as HIV, Zika virus, and COVID-19. Dr. Ferraro holds a dual BA in Biology and Psychology from Johns Hopkins University, an MPH with emphasis in Epidemiology from George Washington University, and a PhD in Health and Behavioral Sciences with specialization in Social Epidemiology from the University of Colorado at Denver. She has published in *Morbidity and Mortality Weekly Report*, *Pediatrics*, *International Health*, and *Vaccines*.

Deborah Finn-Romero, DNP, RN, PHN, PACT, is an assistant professor in the School of Nursing at Sacramento State, teaching in the prelicensure, RN-BSN and graduate programs. She specializes in cardiac, oncology, and infusion/intravenous nursing care; Social Determinants of Health (SDOH); cultural humility; ethics; leadership; and public policy. Dr. Finn-Romero is an inaugural member of the National League for Nursing's SDOH Leadership Academy. As an active advocate of health equity in all levels of nursing and health care equity, she participates as a member in the American Nurses Association/California's Racism in Nursing Academia workgroup and serves as an ANA mentor. Dr. Finn-Romero has published on interprofessional community partnerships focused on improving health outcomes for vulnerable populations. She has presented at Duquesne University's McGinley-Rice Symposium on working with individuals experiencing chronic homelessness and at the NLN Summit on the integration of implicit bias curriculum for prelicensure nursing students.

Melissa Hinds, MSN, RN, is the Associate Director of Health and Technology and Director of Online Assistance Unit at the Center for Practice Innovations (CPI). Melissa Hinds is a registered nurse who oversees and develops curriculum, coordinates projects, and the implementation activities for the System Transformation initiatives. She contributes health care knowledge across CPI activities and products and ensures that CPI's technology platform runs smoothly to meet the Center's increasing needs internally and with our external partners. Ms. Hinds's interest is in changing health care systems. Her primary focus is educating, training, and supporting the behavioral health workforce in clinical core competencies and integrated health care across the lifespan. She is interested in identifying and disseminating effective interventions in psychotic disorders, especially first-episode psychosis, and how we can use technology to reduce the burden of psychotic disorders in resource-poor settings. She works to adapt and teach education strategies for diverse learners and adopt effective evidence-based practices in academic and clinical health care settings to provide the best care for culturally diverse populations and inform nursing research. In her role, she works to develop more integrated care and interprofessional content to help the nurses and other clinicians statewide. In addition to her work with CPI, Ms. Hinds is an adjunct lecturer and clinical instructor at the City University of New York–Bronx Community College and a nursing peer mentor at the City University of New York–School for Professional Studies.

Megan L. Jester, PhD, RN, AHN-BC, is an assistant professor at The University of Oklahoma Health Sciences Fran and Earl Ziegler College of Nursing in Oklahoma City, Oklahoma, where she teaches in the BSN, DNP, and PhD programs. She also serves as a mentor for senior capstone projects at the Stephenson School of Biomedical Engineering on The University of Oklahoma Norman campus. Dr. Jester's clinical experience is in the areas of medical-surgical nursing, postoperative care, mental health, and school nursing. Her research interests examine school-based health promotion in children through the influence of the built environment and mindfulness-based interventions on autonomic function and well-being indicators via community-based participatory collaborations with urban schools. Dr. Jester is board-certified in advanced holistic nursing and has published and presented on innovative active learning experiences, mindfulness-based interventions and autonomic function, and the social and structural determinants of health in school-age children and across nursing curricula.

Sara K. Kaylor, EdD, RN, CNE, is an associate professor at The University of Alabama Capstone College of Nursing, Tuscaloosa Alabama, where she has taught in the BSN and EdD programs for 12 years. Her clinical experience consists of trauma/surgical intensive care nursing. Dr. Kaylor has expertise in curriculum development and evaluation, test item construction and analysis, and professional development. She is active in the National League for Nursing where she currently serves as a Commission for Nursing Education Accreditation (CNEA) site visitor. She is a past scholar in the Social Determinants of Health and Social Policy Change Leadership Academy, sponsored by the NLN and Walden University. Dr. Kaylor is credentialed as a certified nurse educator.

Claire MnKinley Yoder, PhD, RN, CNE, is an assistant professor and program director of the BSN program at University of Portland in Portland, Oregon, where she has taught in the BSN and DNP programs. Her 19 years of teaching experience include undergraduate and graduate teaching in the areas of pediatrics, community and population health, global health, chronic illness, and school nursing. Dr. McKinley Yoder has expertise and has presented both nationally and internationally in the areas of academic-practice partnerships, global health, curriculum development and evaluation, outcomes of school nursing practice, and nursing education. Dr. McKinley Yoder has practiced in the United States, Rwanda, Malawi, and Mexico.

Phyllis D. Morgan, PhD, FNP-BC, CNE, FAANP, is the first PhD in nursing graduate from Hampton University, and first PhD nursing graduate from a Historically Black College/University. Dr. Morgan completed a postdoctoral fellowship at The Johns Hopkins University School of Nursing focused on Health Disparities research. Dr. Morgan is a highly regarded nurse educator, nurse researcher, and nurse practitioner. She is Senior

Core Faculty for the Nurse Practitioner Program at Walden University College of Nursing. She is a Fellow of the American Association of Nurse Practitioners, and a member of several professional nursing organizations. Dr. Morgan was accepted in the first cohort for the National League for Nursing and Walden University College of Nursing Social Determinants of Health & Social Change Leadership Institute. Her research focuses on Social Determinants of Health and Social Change (SDOH) and partnerships with Historically Black Colleges/Universities to prepare students to address SDOH.

Jannyse Tapp, DNP, FNP-BC, is an assistant professor at Vanderbilt University School of Nursing. She is a faculty member in the Family Nurse Practitioner (FNP) Program. Additionally, she serves as the Nurse Midwifery (NM)/Family Nurse Practitioner Dual Student Coordinator. Dr. Tapp's professional journey is driven by a profound commitment to addressing social and structural determinants of health, reducing health disparities, and promoting health equity. Reflecting this passion, she assumes the role of Project Director (PD/PI) for the Collaborative Academic-Practice (CAP) Program, a transformative initiative established under the HRSA-funded Advanced Nursing Education Workforce (ANEW) grant. She also serves as a facilitator for the Poverty Simulation, an experiential learning activity that exposes participants to the realities of poverty. Most recently, Dr. Tapp practiced at a clinic providing care to underserved and vulnerable populations in Nashville. She was accepted into the National League for Nursing/Walden University Social Determinants of Health and Social Change Leadership Academy's inaugural cohort, further solidifying her position as a leader in nursing education, health care, and social determinants of health.

Foreword

"Of all the forms of inequality, injustice in health is the most shocking and inhumane."
—Martin Luther King Jr.

The roots of health inequities are multilayered, complex, and pervasive. They affect everyone, having corollaries that extend beyond generations. To fully understand health inequities, one must recognize the social and structural barriers that create and prolong these disparities. Unfortunately, health care professionals are often not equipped with the requisite knowledge and skills to effectively influence system and policy changes to mitigate the consequences of social and structural determinants of health (SSDH) and to ultimately improve health care and life outcomes.

Although health care workers are strategically poised to play this key role in promoting health equity, mitigating inequity requires intentional education, organizational support, and competence in effectively strategizing policy changes. This comprehensive and thoughtful book provides valuable resources for educators, administrators, and practitioners within the health care professions and beyond, and offers opportunities to employ a continuous systematic evaluation to advance the work of social justice. The collective work deliberately aligns with the National League for Nursing's core value of "Diversity and Inclusion: Affirming the uniqueness of and differences among persons, ideas, values, and ethnicities" by underscoring the critical connection between individuals, families, and communities in shaping health outcomes.

As the editors of this book, Drs. Sandra Davis and Andrea Lindell have strategically curated a compendium of evidence about social and structural determinants of health from the participants in the NLN/Walden University College of Nursing Institute for Social Determinants of Health and Social Change Leadership Academy. This collection offers an exceptional framework for self-reflection, discovery, and engagement, and considers the call to action outlined in *The Future of Nursing 2020–2030: Charting a Path to Achieve Health Equity*. The shared work explores current and relevant information on how social factors—such as wealth, education, neighborhood characteristics, and racism—and factors such as power and social values shape health and health inequities. This book provides the support to help guide health care professionals through an introspective and transformational journey that challenges their existing paradigm and asks them to consider the upstream factors or underlying causes of health disparities that shape the downstream factors of access to health care, personal life choices, social risk factors, and living conditions. The profound content prompts the reader to strengthen their capacity and commitment to advancing health equity and to become effective influencers, change agents, and leaders.

I commend and congratulate the editors of this work for being bold and passionate in their commitment to having the necessary crucial conversations about the impact of social and structural determinants of health. This book poses a question to the individual, at the personal level: "What is my commitment, my drive, and my motivation to do this important work?" It is an important query that all health care workers should contemplate. I am honored to recommend this work by the outstanding editors and the participants in the NLN/Walden Leadership Academy as they strive to advance the health of the nation and the global community.

Patricia A. Sharpnack, DNP, RN, CNE, NEA-BC, FAAN, ANEF
Chair, National League for Nursing
Dean and Strawbridge Professor
Ursuline College, Breen School of Nursing and Health Professions
Pepper Pike, Ohio

Preface

Health equity, both as a concept and a vision, is not new—it is centuries old. As a vision, it is the North Star for nurses and health professionals who strive for everyone to have a fair opportunity to live their healthiest life possible. As a concept, it is complex and multidimensional, with the terms "health disparity," "health inequality," and "health inequity" often used interchangeably to measure progress toward the attainment of the highest level of health for all people. Notably, the term "heath inequity" is used throughout this book. "Health inequity" is defined as the *systematic, unnecessary, and avoidable differences in health or the major socially determined influences on health between groups of people who have different relative positions in social hierarchies based on wealth, power, or prestige, which can be shaped by policies* (Braveman et al., 2018; Whitehead, 1992; WHO, 2018). The intentional use of the term "health inequity" underscores the progression in understanding, recognizing, and acknowledging the critical importance of social and structural determinants of health in advancing health equity. Addressing social conditions that disproportionately impact health has long been a cornerstone of nursing practice. However, new to the profession is an upstream perspective that focuses on the inextricable connection between systems and structures, policy and politics, and structural racism as drivers of inequity.

After nearly four decades of the promotion of health equity in the United States, gaps in health care delivery and health outcomes are wide, persistent, and increasing. Our 40-year timeline of advancing health equity consists of gaps in evidence and inconsistencies in action. In 1899, W. E. B. DuBois described how social determinants, racism, and systemic and structural inequities impact health in the United States (Du Bois, 1899). However, the concept of social determinants of health (SDH) did not gain momentum until 2010 with the release of Healthy People 2020. It was not until 2020, with the murder of George Floyd and the disproportionate impact of COVID-19, that serious attention was given to structural determinants as drivers of health inequities.

SDH are the conditions in which people are born, grow, live, work, and age, and the wider set of forces and systems shaping the conditions of daily life (WHO, 2022). Although the definition of SDH encompasses both social conditions and the wider forces and systems that affect health, the latter part of the definition has often been omitted, considered inconsequential, or not even discussed (Weil, 2021). With the evidence and acknowledgment of structural determinants, including structural racism, as a root cause of health inequity, nurse leaders have an opportunity to actively drive the transformative social change needed to advance health equity.

Nursing leaders often look for the best opportunity to make an impact. Although goals and expected outcomes are planned, the journey is often unplanned. For nurses and other health care professionals in or aspiring to positions to lead the needed transformation in health care, this book serves as a roadmap for taking leadership to a higher level by becoming a creative agent for social change. The contributors to this book were participants in the inaugural NLN/Walden University College of Nursing Institute for Social Determinants of Health and Social Change Leadership Academy. Through meaningful content, case studies, practical exemplars, and challenging thoughts to consider, the authors provide a setting for discovery, analysis, and application through the often-untapped lens of systems, structures, and root causes. This book is a valuable resource that allows the reader to go from the current reality—of their impact as a leader in advancing health equity—to the possibility of an intentional and purposefully profound impact by making critical connections to the inextricable role of systems, structures, and root causes of health inequity.

Sandra Davis, PhD, DPM, ACNP-BC, FAANP
Andrea Lindell, PhD, RN, ANEF

References

Braveman, P., Arkin, E., Orleans, T., Proctor, D., Acker, J., & Plough, A. (2018). What is health equity? *Behavioral Science & Policy*, 4(1), 1–14.

Du Bois, W. E. B. (1899). *The Philadelphia Negro: A social study*. The University of Pennsylvania Press.

Weil, A. (2021, June 3). The Social Determinants of Death. *Health Affairs*. https://www.healthaffairs.org/do/10.1377/forefront.20200603.831955/

Whitehead, M. (1992). The concepts and principles of equity and health. *International Journal of Health Services*, 22(3), 429–445. https://www.jstor.org/stable/45131055

World Health Organization (WHO). (2018, February 22). Health inequities and their causes. https://www.who.int/news-room/facts-in-pictures/detail/health-inequities-and-their-causes#:~:text=Health%20inequities%20are%20systematic%20differences,shows%20their%20cost%20to%20society.

World Health Organization (WHO). (2022). Social Determinants of Health. https://www.who.int/health-topics/social-determinants-of-health#tab=tab_1

Contents

List of Figures, Tables, and Boxes

LIST OF BOXES

Introduction

Megan L. Jester, PhD, RN, AHN-BC
Aimee Ferraro, PhD, MPH
Deborah Finn-Romero, DNP, RN, PHN, PACT
Sara K. Kaylor, EdD, RN, CNE

This book focuses on the interconnectedness between the individual, the family, and the community, and how social, structural, political, environmental, educational, and economic mechanisms influence health. Understanding the social and structural drivers of health is foundational to achieving health equity. Moreover, recognizing the influence of systems, structures, policies, practices, and norms on health inequities is essential. Structural competency is the ability to recognize systems, institutional norms, policies, and practices that produce unjust health conditions (Metzl & Hansen, 2014). Nurses and other health care professionals committed to providing structurally competent care must actively engage in a continuous process of learning, self-reflection, collaboration, and advocacy. These efforts are essential in addressing the multifaceted social and structural determinants of health (SSDH) that contribute to health inequities.

PROBLEM AND BACKGROUND

The COVID-19 pandemic highlighted the persistent and growing inequities in health care access, outcomes, and quality, particularly among historically excluded and underrepresented groups. Health care and nursing professionals face complex and interconnected health care delivery challenges, further compounded by systemic issues such as structural racism, political conflicts, social unrest, and climate change. Effectively addressing these challenges necessitates interdisciplinary collaboration and a keen focus on SSDH.

The SSDH comprise a range of economic, social, structural, and environmental factors that significantly influence our overall health and well-being. Structural factors, within a sociopolitical context, drive poverty, health literacy, housing stability, food access, and health insurance status, all of which profoundly impact both our physical and mental health. Although nurses and health care professionals have traditionally addressed these factors, an upstream approach that focuses on systems and structures, policy and politics, and deep-rooted historical causes of inequities has not been sufficiently integrated into educational and practice environments.

HOW THIS BOOK IS ORGANIZED

This book offers a comprehensive guide to integrating SSDH into nursing and interdisciplinary programs, curricula, and practice. It presents content, practical exemplars, and challenging questions to assist with the integration of SSDH to educate not only nursing leaders, but all health care professionals, ultimately working toward reducing health inequities. The book is organized into chapters on the following topics: curriculum, practice, partnerships, dissemination and research, and administration and leadership. Each chapter provides an in-depth look at the key concepts related to SSDH and suggests detailed strategies for incorporating SSDH into higher education curricula and practice.

This book follows the *Social Determinants of Health* framework established by the World Health Organization (WHO) in 2008 and adopted by Healthy People 2020 and 2030. This framework identifies five major domains critical to understanding the upstream factors that influence health inequities: education access and quality, economic stability, health care access and quality, neighborhood and built environment, and social and community context. It is important to note that Healthy People 2030 identifies structural racism and systemic bias as social determinants of health. The five domains are inextricably connected to these concepts, with each impacting the others.

Education Access and Quality

Education refers to the level of formal learning achieved by an individual (Krieger, 2001; WHO, 2008). Education provides individuals with knowledge and skills to make informed decisions about their health, enhances critical thinking abilities, and fosters a sense of empowerment. In addition, education is closely intertwined with socioeconomic status and employment opportunities, collectively exerting a profound influence on one's overall quality of life (USDHHS & ODPHP, 2020). Structural racism, economics, politics, and policies are structural determinants that impact educational systems.

Economic Stability

Employment and working conditions encompass various aspects of one's job, including elements such as job stability, income, workload, and exposure to workplace hazards (Krieger, 2001; WHO, 2008). Gainful employment not only provides financial security but also enhances psychological well-being by fostering social integration and inclusion. Conversely, unstable employment and unsafe workplaces can contribute to stress, workplace injuries, and the development of chronic health problems (Marmot, 2004). Employment and economic stability must be viewed within the historical and contemporary sociopolitical contexts of the United States, with a focus on structural racism.

Health Care Access and Quality

Access to health care services refers to the ease with which individuals can obtain essential medical care when required (WHO, 2008). This encompasses factors such as the physical proximity to health care facilities, affordability of services, and the availability of health insurance. Structural barriers to health care access, such as inadequate health care infrastructure in underserved areas, can disproportionately impact historically excluded underrepresented populations and play a significant role in contributing to health inequities (USDHHS & ODPHP, 2020).

Neighborhood and Built Environment

Housing and neighborhood conditions encompass both the physical and social environment in which individuals reside (Krieger, 2001; WHO, 2008). Substandard housing conditions, a lack of affordable housing options, and exposure to environmental hazards, such as pollution or crime, can have adverse effects on health. It is critical to analyze and address the structural drivers, both historic and contemporary, of these conditions. For example, redlining and racial segregation must be understood and discussed. Conversely, access to green spaces, recreational facilities, and community resources contributes to the creation of healthier communities (USDHHS & ODPHP, 2020).

Social and Community Context

Social support and social networks comprise the relationships, friendships, and family connections that offer emotional, instrumental, and informational assistance (Berkman et al., 2000; Krieger, 2001). Strong social ties play a vital role in promoting mental and emotional well-being, serving as a buffer against stress, and facilitating access to valuable resources. Conversely, social isolation and a lack of social support are linked with adverse health outcomes, including mental health disorders and chronic illnesses (Berkman & Syme, 1979). It is imperative to examine how structural racism is embedded in systems, laws, policies, practices, and attitudes.

Structural Racism

Structural racism is a concept defined as the myriad ways in which societies perpetuate racial discrimination through mutually reinforcing inequitable systems (Bailey et al., 2017; Egede & Walker, 2020). Examples of these systems include mass incarceration, historic practices such as redlining or residential segregation, and education policies (Egede et al., 2022). Structural racism operates at multiple levels, profoundly impacting individuals and communities. Addressing structural racism is essential for achieving racial equity and justice.

THE AUDIENCE FOR THIS BOOK

This book serves as a valuable educational resource for educators, administrators, and practitioners within the health care professions. *Educators* can utilize this book as a guide to develop and teach courses focused on SSDH to health care students. It offers practical insights to help educators design effective educational strategies that seamlessly integrate SSDH into existing curricula, equipping students to address the social challenges that significantly impact their patients' health outcomes. *Administrators* can leverage this book to foster holistic and sustainable infrastructures, policies, and workflows, with a primary focus on identifying patients who require referrals for intervention and evaluating outcomes related to SSDH. *Practitioners*, too, can benefit from this resource, gaining a deeper understanding of how research and evidence-based practices related to SSDH can assist in identifying patients with unmet needs. Furthermore, it provides guidance on referring these patients to appropriate community resources and support services. The book also aids practitioners in the development and implementation of policies and guidelines that facilitate the integration of SSDH into health care practice.

MULTIDISCIPLINARY APPROACH

The most pressing health care and societal inequities cannot be resolved by any single discipline alone. In this book, we employ exemplars to explore SSDH from the perspectives of public health, nursing, and medicine. This approach serves to illustrate the imperative for interdisciplinary action and collaboration in our efforts to advance health equity.

CHALLENGES AND CHANGE AT THE INDIVIDUAL LEVEL

Although collective action is necessary, the authors also realize that change starts at the individual level and is uniquely personal. The "Challenging Thoughts to Consider" section at the end of each chapter provides the reader with opportunities to think about ways to apply the chapter content while examining one's individual drive and motivation for wanting to lead this needed transformation in health care.

OPERATIONAL DEFINITIONS AND KEY TERMS

Cultural Humility

Cultural humility is an approach developed to address power imbalances between health care providers and patients. It encourages providers to engage in self-reflection, thereby increasing self-awareness and facilitating the transformation of biases and attitudes toward diverse populations (Tervalon & Murray-Garcia, 1998). Cultural humility differs from cultural competence, because it does not solely focus on acquiring theoretical knowledge about a cultural group as a monolith, but rather emphasizes the importance of addressing the biases held by the provider. Cultural humility necessitates a lifelong commitment to introspection and strives to create more equal partnerships within the provider–patient relationship (Tervalon & Murray-Garcia, 1998).

Environmental Justice

Environmental justice embodies the principle of ensuring equitable and meaningful participation for all individuals, irrespective of their race, color, national origin, identity, or income, in the formulation, execution, and enforcement of environmental laws, regulations, and policies (Annie E. Casey Foundation, 2021; U.S. Department of Energy, 2023). It is the idea that all people have the right to live and thrive in healthy environments with equal protections (American Public Health Association, 2024). This commitment to fairness entails that no community should bear an undue burden of adverse environmental impacts stemming from industrial, municipal, or commercial activities and the implementation of federal, state, and local regulations and policies (Anne E. Casey Foundation, 2021).

Health Equity

Health equity refers to the fundamental principle of ensuring that all individuals have an equal opportunity to attain their highest level of health (Braveman et al., 2017). Achieving health equity involves addressing systemic and structural barriers that contribute to health inequities among different populations. It acknowledges that attaining equal health outcomes may necessitate the mitigation of social, economic, and environmental determinants of health. Additionally, health equity involves the implementation of targeted interventions aimed at reducing unjust health inequities and promoting fairness in health care access and outcomes (Braveman et al., 2018).

Health Inequity

Conversely, health inequity is the systematic, unnecessary, and avoidable differences in health between groups of people who have different relative positions in social hierarchies based on wealth, structural racism, or power, all of which can be shaped by policy (Braveman at al., 2018; Whitehead, 1992).

Implicit Bias

Implicit bias, also referred to as implicit prejudice or implicit attitude, is an unconscious negative attitude toward a specific social group. It is believed to be shaped by personal experiences and formed through learned associations between certain qualities and social categories, such as race or gender. Individuals may be influenced by their implicit biases in their perceptions and behaviors even though they are unaware of holding such biases. Implicit bias is a component of implicit social cognition, which encompasses the phenomenon that perceptions, attitudes, and stereotypes can operate without conscious intention or endorsement (American Psychological Association [APA], 2022).

Racial Justice

Racial justice constitutes the systematic equitable treatment of individuals across all racial demographics, targeting structural inequities that affect social determinants of health, and facilitating equal opportunities and outcomes for all members of society (Annie E. Casey Foundation, 2021). This approach ensures that every individual can achieve their optimal health status, free from the constraints of racial, ethnic, or community-related inequities.

Racism

Racism is a system of structuring opportunity and assigning value based on the social interpretation of how one looks, which is the social construct we call race. This unfairly disadvantages some individuals and communities, unfairly advantages other individuals and communities, and saps the strength of the whole society through the waste of human resources (Jones, 2018).

Social Justice

In the context of health, social justice emphasizes that achieving optimal health is a societal responsibility rooted in principles of justice and human rights (Braveman et al., 2011). The primary objective of social justice in health care is to eliminate inequities in both access to health care and its quality, with a particular focus on underrepresented communities. This concept underscores the significance of implementing policies that prioritize health equity, aiming to reduce systemic inequalities and to foster fairness in health care.

Social and Structural Determinants of Health

Social and structural determinants of health (SSDH) encompass the multifaced factors that play a pivotal role in shaping health outcomes and contribute to health inequities within populations (Krieger, 2001; WHO, 2008; WHO, 2010; Wilkinson & Marmot, 2003). The SSDH are defined as conditions in which people are born, grow, live, work, and age, **and the wider set of forces and systems shaping the conditions of daily life** (WHO, 2022a). Wider forces include economics, development agendas, cultural and social norms, historical and contemporary policies, and political systems, and laws, all of which influence the distribution of money, power, and resources (WHO, 2022b).

Structural Competency

Structural competency is a framework for conceptualizing and addressing the systems, institutional norms, practices, and policies that produce inequitable and unjust health situations and conditions (Davis & O'Brien, 2020; Metzl & Hansen, 2014). Concepts central to structural competency are structural inequity, structural racism, and structural stigma (Metzl & Hansen, 2014).

CONCLUSION AND CALL TO ACTION

This book underscores the vital interconnectedness between individuals, families, and communities in shaping health outcomes, while highlighting the profound impact of social, structural, political, environmental, educational, and economic factors on health. It emphasizes that health care professionals—particularly nurses—who are dedicated to providing structurally competent care must engage in an ongoing process of learning, self-reflection, collaboration, and advocacy. These collective endeavors are crucial for addressing the complex web of SSDH that underlies health inequities. Throughout our exploration of SSDH, we introduce key terms—such as structural racism, implicit bias, income inequality, and social support—which lay the groundwork for comprehending the content within this book. Recognizing that the most pressing health care and societal challenges transcend disciplinary boundaries, we employ a case-based approach to examine SSDH through the lenses of public health, nursing, and medicine. This methodology highlights the necessity for interdisciplinary cooperation and collective action as we lead the advancement of health equity.

Challenging Thoughts to Consider

1. Why is it important to personally reflect on one's experience with the definitions and key terms mentioned above? What do these definitions and terms look like in the organizations that you lead?
2. Discuss the value of utilizing structural competency as a framework for addressing health and social inequities.

References

American Psychological Association. (2022). Topic. Implicit Bias. https://www.apa.org/topics/implicit-bias

American Public Health Association. (2024). Environmental Justice. https://www.apha.org/Topics-and-Issues/Environmental-Health/Environmental-Justice

Annie E. Casey Foundation. (2021). Equity, Inclusion, and Other Racial Justice Definitions. https://www.aecf.org/blog/racial-justice-definitions

Bailey, Z. D., Krieger, N., Agénor, M., Graves, J., Linos, N., & Bassett, M. T. (2017). Structural racism and health inequities in the USA: evidence and interventions. *Lancet*, *389*(10077), 1453–1463.

Bailey, Z. D., Feldman, J. M., & Bassett, M. T. (2021). How structural racism works-racist policies as a root cause of U.S. racial health inequities. *New England Journal of Medicine*, *384*(8), 768–773. https://doi.org/10.1056/NEJMms2025396

Berkman, L. F., Kawachi, I., & Glymour, M. M. (Eds.). (2000). *Social epidemiology*. Oxford University Press.

Berkman, L. F., & Syme, S. L. (1979). Social networks, host resistance, and mortality: A nine-year follow-up study of Alameda County residents. *American Journal of Epidemiology*, *109*(2), 186–204. https://doi.org/10.1093/oxfordjournals.aje.a112674

Braveman, P., Arkin, E., Orleans, T., Proctor, D., Acker, J., & Plough, A. (2018). What is health equity? *Behavioral Science & Policy*, *4*(1), 1–14.

Braveman, P., Arkin, E., Orleans, T., Proctor, D., & Plough, A. (2017). *What is health equity? And what difference does a definition make?* Robert Wood Johnson Foundation.

Braveman, P. A., Kumanyika, S., Fielding, J., Laveist, T., Borrell, L. N., Manderscheid, R., & Troutman, A. (2011). Health disparities and health equity: the issue is justice. *American Journal of Public Health*, *101*(Suppl 1), S149–S155.

Davis, S., & O'Brien, A.-M. (2020). Let's talk about racism: Building structural competency in nursing. *Academic Medicine*, *95*(12S), S58–S65.

Egede, L. E, Walker, R. J., Linde, S., Campbell, J. A., Dawson, A. Z., Williams, J. S., & Ozieh, M. N. (2022). Nonmedical interventions for type 2 diabetes: Evidence, actionable strategies, and policy opportunities. *Health Affairs*, *41*(2). https://doi.org/10.1377/hlthaff.2022.00236

Egede, L. E., & Walker, R. J. (2020). Structural racism, social risk factors, and Covid-19—a dangerous convergence for Black Americans. *New England Journal of Medicine*, *383*(12), e77.

Jones, C. P. (2018). Toward the science and practice of anti-racism: Launching a national campaign against racism. *Ethnicity and Disease*, *28*(Suppl 1), 231–234.

Krieger N. (2001). A glossary for social epidemiology. *Journal of Epidemiology and Community Health*, *55*(10), 693–700. https://doi.org/10.1136/jech.55.10.693

Marmot M. (2004). *The status syndrome: How your social standing affects your health and life expectancy*. Bloomsbury.

Metzl, J. M., & Hansen, H. (2014). Structural competency: Theorizing a new medical engagement with stigma and inequality. *Social Science & Medicine, 103*, 126–133.

Tervalon, M., & Murray-Garcia, J. (1998). Cultural humility versus cultural competence: A critical distinction in defining physician training outcomes in multicultural education. *Journal of Health Care for the Poor and Underserved, 9*(2), 117–125. https://doi.org/10.1353/hpu.2010.0233

U.S. Department of Energy (USDE) Office of Legacy Management (OLM). (2023). *What is environmental justice?* https://www.energy.gov/lm/what-environmental-justice

U.S. Department of Health and Human Services (USDHHS) & Office of Disease Prevention and Health Promotion (ODPHP). (2020). *Healthy People 2030*. https://health.gov/healthypeople/objectives-and-data/social-determinants-health

Whitehead, M. (1992). The concepts and principles of equity and health. *International Journal of Health Services, 22*(3), 429–445. https://www.jstor.org/stable/45131055

Wilkinson, R. G., & Marmot, M. (Eds.). (2003). *Social determinants of health: The solid facts*. World Health Organization. https://apps.who.int/iris/bitstream/handle/10665/326568/9789289013710-eng.pdf?sequence=1&isAllowed=y

World Health Organization Commission on Social Determinants of Health. (2008). *Closing the gap in a generation: Health equity through action on the social determinants of health*. https://www.who.int/teams/social-determinants-of-health/equity-and-health/commission-on-social-determinants-of-health

World Health Organization. (2010a). *A conceptual framework for action on the social determinants of health*. https://apps.who.int/iris/bitstream/handle/10665/44489/?sequence=1

World Health Organization (WHO). (2022a). *Social Determinants of Health*. https://www.who.int/health-topics/social-determinants-of-health#tab=tab_1

World Health Organization (WHO). (2022b). *Taking action on the social determinants of health*. https://www.who.int/western-pacific/activities/taking-action-on-the-social-determinants-of-health

Yearby, R. (2020). Structural racism and health disparities: Reconfiguring the social determinants of health framework to include the root cause. *Journal of Law, Medicine & Ethics, 48*(3), 518–552.

Curriculum: Developing Future Health Care Professionals

Sara K. Kaylor, EdD, RN, CNE
Aimee Ferraro, PhD, MPH
Claire McKinley Yoder, PhD, RN, CNE

INTRODUCTION

The health care industry is constantly evolving, and with it, the need for competent and compassionate health care providers. However, becoming a skilled health care provider requires more than just technical knowledge and clinical skills, and the importance of addressing social and structural determinants of health (SSDH) in health care education and practice cannot be overstated. In recent years, there has been a growing recognition of the crucial impact that SSDH play in shaping the health outcomes of individuals and communities. Understanding, assessing, and addressing these factors is essential for the development of structural competence in our future health care practitioners. In this chapter, we will delve into the critical importance of developing and evaluating SSDH curriculum, as well as exploring a range of educational strategies that are essential to prepare students who are transitioning into health care provider roles to meet the diverse needs of their patients and communities.

Values and Alignment

Preparing the next generation of health care practitioners with the skills and attitudes to address SDH and move society toward health equity is critical work. All members of the NLN SDH Academy were also faculty engaged in this important work and the Academy extended the knowledge, leadership, and advocacy skills necessary to transform curricula.

Chapter Objectives

Upon completion of this chapter, the learner will be able to:

1. Discuss the importance of addressing SSDH in health care education and practice to develop structurally competent health care professionals.

2. Analyze the development and evaluation of SSDH curriculum as a means of promoting the health care provider competency in addressing SSDH.

3. Evaluate a range of educational strategies, such as didactic lectures, case studies, simulations, and experiential learning activities, for teaching SSDH to health care students.

4. Identify barriers and challenges in implementing SSDH curriculum and educational strategies in health care education and practice.

5. Propose solutions and recommendations for effectively addressing SSDH in health care education and practice to promote health equity.

DEVELOPMENT OF A SOCIAL DETERMINANTS OF HEALTH CURRICULUM

In 2008, the World Health Organization (WHO) released the final report of the Commission on Social Determinants of Health, which established a framework for promoting health equity and fostered a global movement to achieve it (WHO, 2008). In the following decade, several leading health organizations issued calls to action to incorporate SSDH in the education and training of health professionals, including the National Academies of Sciences, Engineering, and Medicine (NASEM) in 2016 and the National League for Nursing (NLN) in 2019. NASEM (2016) recommended that educational organizations "foster an enabling environment that supports and values the integration of the framework's principles into their mission, culture, and work" (p. 91). NLN (2019) added that universities must use evidence-based approaches to teaching and learning strategies related to SSDH, thread SSDH education throughout the program of learning in varied educational settings (e.g., classroom, practice settings, and simulation-learning environments), and create partnerships with community agencies to intentionally expose students to real-world experiences related to SSDH (p. 6). In other words, teaching one course on SSDH is not sufficient. Universities must establish supportive infrastructure, comprehensive curricula, longitudinal training, and evidence-based research on SSDH to make a significant impact on health equity.

THE ROLE OF CURRICULA IN DEVELOPING STRUCTURALLY COMPETENT HEALTH CARE PROFESSIONALS

A well-developed curriculum serves as a structured and comprehensive educational roadmap for educators by outlining the scope and sequence of learning experiences, content, and activities that students will engage in within their specific educational program. One of the key challenges facing health profession educators is re-envisioning the curriculum to prepare structurally competent practitioners. These future practitioners must be capable of adapting to an ever-changing and evolving health care system, while also being empowered to challenge the status quo and act as agents of change in combating the systemic and structural racism prevalent within the health care system.

Curricula focused on SSDH are timely and important. Historically, health care education has emphasized biomedical factors as the primary cause of disease and disease processes, neglecting social, economic, and environmental factors that can significantly impact individual differences, preferences, lifestyle factors, patterns, and behaviors. As the importance of SSDH in shaping health outcomes has become more widely recognized, health care education has shifted to incorporate more training on these factors. Curriculum focused on SSDH ensures that future health care practitioners have the knowledge, attitudes, and skills they need to competently address these factors in their practice, promoting more comprehensive and patient-centered care.

Incorporating SSDH into curricula is also essential for promoting health equity, as inequities related to SSDH are well documented. Health care practitioners who are equipped to address these factors can work toward promoting health equity by providing care that is tailored to the specific needs of their patients and communities. Lastly, evaluation of SSDH curriculum is also critical to ensure its effectiveness and to identify areas for improvement. Assessment strategies, such as pre- and post-tests, surveys, and focus groups, can be used to evaluate the impact of SSDH curriculum on learners' knowledge, attitudes, and skills.

Curricular Scanning and Mapping

In today's rapidly changing world, education must adapt and be responsive to the evolving demands of society. As such, a curriculum that effectively prepares health care practitioners for the challenges and opportunities of the future requires a proactive approach from faculty members, who serve as architects of the educational experience, responsible for shaping the knowledge and skills imparted to students. Several strategies exist that enable faculty to scan and forecast the forces and issues influential to curriculum designs, as well as map or "crosswalk" existing curricula to assess gaps and opportunities. Regularly assessing internal and external factors allows faculty to identify emerging needs and challenges, which can then be incorporated into new subject matter, teaching methodologies, and relevant experiences in the curriculum. Actively seeking input from various stakeholders (e.g., industry professionals, alumni, and even students themselves) is another important consideration for incorporating diverse perspectives and ensuring that the curricula align with the needs of both the job market and society at large.

Strategic forecasting and planning are crucial skills for deans, administrators, and faculty alike, especially when integrating concepts of SSDH into the curriculum for the health professions. One component of this process is environmental scanning, which involves the monitoring and evaluating of information from various sources to identify threats and opportunities, as well as strengths and weaknesses (Decker et al., 2005; Layman et al., 2010; Suh et al., 2004; Veltri, 2020). The goal of environmental scanning is to empower leaders and faculty to recognize general trends and events affecting health care, higher education, and more specifically, health profession education (Veltri, 2020).

When integrating SSDH into the curriculum, environmental scanning takes on a transformative element, enabling faculty to be both reactive and proactive in their approach (Veltri, 2020). By keenly observing significant trends (reactive), faculty can proactively shape the future direction of health professions education, ensuring that it addresses the profound impact of social determinants on health outcomes. Environmental scanning, thus, becomes an indispensable tool for health profession educators, helping them stay ahead of emerging challenges and seize opportunities for innovation. By maintaining a pulse of the ever-changing landscape of health care, educators can create a curriculum that fosters a deeper understanding of social factors—influencing health inequities—and equips future health care practitioners with the knowledge, skills, and structural competence to address these inequities effectively.

External Factors Influencing Curricula

Externally, faculty must be aware of the latest advancements and emerging trends influencing the health care landscape, as well as the broader societal issues currently shaping the profession, including health inequities, systemic racism, and the profound influence of SSDH. The concept of "environmental turbulence" (Layman et al., 2010, p. 11) encompasses the constant and often unpredictable changes impacting health care, driven by various factors, such as advancements in medical technology, evolving health care policies, and fluctuating funding and resources. State, national, and global economic landscapes also exert significant influence on the health care industry, impacting funding models, reimbursement mechanisms, and the overall accessibility of health care services. An increasingly diverse and multicultural society also impacts health care practices and patient interactions, necessitating cultural awareness, humility, and sensitivity among health care professionals. In accounting for these and other external factors, faculty play a pivotal role in the curriculum and its development, by emphasizing the importance of health equity, guiding students to recognize the interconnectedness between social factors and health outcomes, and fostering an inclusive and antiracist learning environment. These efforts aim to dismantle biases and promote structural competence in health care practitioners.

State and national political climates also significantly influence public institutions of higher education. The impact of this influence was evident in early 2023 when several Republican-controlled states in the U.S. proposed bills to remove diversity, equity, and inclusion (DEI) initiatives from their state colleges. During that time, at least two dozen bills were introduced in 15 states, seeking to undo DEI efforts through funding reductions or restrictions on how race and identity are discussed and handled in educational settings (Marijolovic, 2023). Adding to the complexity, on June 29, 2023, the U.S. Supreme Court ruled in a 6-3 decision that race-conscious admission practices are unconstitutional, thus ending decades of support for considering race as a factor in college admission decisions. In response to this ruling, the National Association of Diversity Officers in Higher Education (NADOHE, 2023) argued that it presents yet another obstacle for students seeking equitable access to the opportunities that a college degree offers, such as higher earnings and lower rates of unemployment. Removing racial considerations from college admissions serves to oppress people of color and places the responsibility on individual colleges to develop race-neutral programs to advance their diversity efforts. The NLN (2023) also joined the larger higher education community in disagreeing with the Supreme Court's decision, emphasizing that this ruling jeopardizes public health, precisely at a time when the need for a diverse nursing workforce is paramount for reducing health inequities, addressing SSDH, and promoting excellence in nursing education to advance the health of the nation and the global community. These evolving political issues remain at the forefront for faculty and higher education administrators, as they continuously scan the external environment for influences on the curriculum.

Internal Factors Influencing Curricula

Internal institutional factors, encompassing aspects such as institutional culture, available resources, and organizational capabilities, wield a considerable influence on the student's educational experience. Recognizing the strengths and limitations inherent in the educational system enables faculty to make well-informed decisions about curriculum development and implementation. Introducing a comprehensive curriculum reform hinges on three pivotal factors, explained by Oliver and Hyun (2011) as catalysts for organizational change: financial stability, an appropriate organizational infrastructure, and a shared vision.

A financially secure institution can allocate essential resources to facilitate effective curriculum changes involving facilities, technology, and comprehensive support services for faculty, staff, and students. Budgetary constraints frequently influence the capacity of faculty, deans, and department heads to enact meaningful curriculum changes. These constraints often manifest in two distinct ways. First, a particular specialty course may be perceived as being too expensive or otherwise financially burdensome, thus prompting the provision of a "trimmed down" or condensed version instead, which ultimately diminishes the overall quality of the curriculum change. Secondly, larger class sizes for such specialty courses may alternatively be adopted, thus affecting the type of teaching and learning methodologies to be incorporated (Lachiver & Tardif, 2002; Lemay & Moreau, 2020).

The success of a curriculum transformation is significantly influenced by the institution's overall philosophy and shared vision toward change and the new curriculum. An institutional ethos that acknowledges the value of curriculum change and actively seeks improvement is a driving force for successful transitions (Fullan, 2005; Hargreaves & Fink, 2006; Rudhumbu, 2015). The notion of shared governance and collaboration regarding decision-making is vital for effectively managing the intricate balance between curricular concerns linked to students' academic achievement and the departmental unit's role responsibility within the curriculum (Hyun, 2009; Oliver & Hyun, 2011). Myers (2006) said, "No dean wants to instigate a turf war among faculty members and their guilds, but curricular revisioning almost always leads to such a moment unless a rapprochement can be reached via a faculty's shared vision and understanding of a common mission" (p. 35).

Emphasizing shared governance within the development of an SSDH curriculum cultivates an environment where collaborative decision-making, rooted in mutual respect and effective communication, becomes a cornerstone of curricular change. Involving key stakeholders from diverse backgrounds, including faculty, students, administrators, and community representatives, ensures that a broad spectrum of perspectives, experiences, and expertise contribute to the decision-making process, leading to a curriculum that is holistic, comprehensive, and responsive to the complexities of health and well-being within diverse communities. Myers (2006) recognizes that when stakeholders collaborate on the evaluation of learning goals associated with the curriculum change, an opportunity for dialogue and critical reflection on major issues is created. As stakeholders collectively assess these goals in the context of SSDH of health, they engage in substantive discussions that delve into the complex interplay between structural, socioeconomic, environmental, and cultural factors in shaping health outcomes, which encourage a deeper understanding of the real-world implications of these determinants, sparking insightful and innovative approaches that can be integrated into the curriculum.

COMPETENCIES FOR HEALTH PROFESSIONS

Health practitioners need to possess a specific level of knowledge, skills, abilities, and behaviors to ensure the delivery of safe, effective, and high-quality care to diverse patient populations. Core competencies serve as a fundamental framework for establishing baseline levels and performance expectations within the roles of such practitioners. Health profession educators hold the responsibility of equipping graduates with the skills needed to meet the established competencies of their discipline. Box 1.1 outlines a set of recommended core competencies that are essential for all health care practitioners, regardless of their specific discipline.

As frontline providers of care, nurses witness firsthand the effects inequities have on patients under their care. In 2021, the NLN Commission for Nursing Education Accreditation (CNEA) released updated *Accreditation Standards for Nursing Education*

BOX 1.1

Core Competencies Needed for Health Care Professionals

Provide patient-centered care—recognize and value patients' diverse characteristics, beliefs, and needs; alleviate pain and distress; ensure consistent and coordinated care; effectively communicate and educate patients; share decision-making and management; and actively promote disease prevention, wellness, and healthy lifestyles, with a focus on both individual and population health.

Work in interdisciplinary teams—work together; communicate effectively; and integrate care within teams to ensure dependable and reliable patient care.

Employ evidence-based practice—integrate the best research findings, clinical expertise, and patient values to provide optimal care, while also engaging in learning and research activities whenever feasible.

Apply quality improvement—recognize care errors and risks; apply fundamental safety design principles; consistently assess care quality based on patient and community needs; and devise and evaluate interventions to enhance care processes and systems, with the goal of enhancing overall quality.

Utilize informatics—utilize information technology to effectively communicate, handle knowledge, prevent errors, and facilitate decision-making.

Source: National Academy of Sciences (NAS, 2003).

Programs, emphasizing the role that a "culture of diversity" plays in all types of nursing programs, from practical/vocational through clinical doctoral education. This is evident in that faculty design program curricula to "create a culture of learning that fosters the human flourishing and professional identity formation of diverse learners through professional and personal growth" (NLN, 2021, p. 32).

These updated CNEA accreditation standards reflect a paradigm shift that has emerged within health profession education, which moves away from an emphasis on culturally competent care only to instead view the delivery of care through the lens of structural competency (Davis & O'Brien, 2020; Metzl & Hansen, 2014) (see Table 1.1; NLN, 2021). The term "structural competence" refers to the capacity of health care

TABLE 1.1

Selected Standards, Quality Indicators, and Interpretive Guidelines for Nursing Education Programs

Standard III: Culture of Excellence and Caring—Faculty	
III-A	The program's faculty is qualified, diverse, and adequate in number to meet program goals. *Interpretive Guidelines:* ➤ Adequate number of faculty with expertise in social determinants of health, population health, health equity, and technological competence to meet the program goals.
Standard IV: Culture of Excellence and Caring—Students	
IV-A	The institution and program provide student services that are student-centered; culturally responsive, inclusive, and readily accessible to all students, including those enrolled in distance education; and guide students through the processes associated with admission, recruitment, retention, progression, graduation, and career planning. Student services are evaluated for effectiveness and ability to satisfactorily meet diverse student needs through a process of continuous quality improvement.
Standard V: Culture of Learning and Diversity—Curriculum and Evaluation Processes	
V-D	The curriculum is up-to-date, dynamic, evidence-based, and reflects current and emerging societal and health care trends and issues, research findings, and contemporary educational practices. *Interpretive Guidelines:* ➤ The curriculum demonstrates evidence of education based on health care quality, social determinants of health, health equity, population health, and ethical practice. ➤ The curriculum demonstrates evidence of education of nurse well-being, resilience, and self-care. ➤ Relevant local, regional, national, and international social and health care trends and issues, and workforce needs are addressed as appropriate within the curriculum and in congruence with the program's mission, goals, values, and expected program outcomes.

Adapted from the National League for Nursing (NLN) Commission for Nursing Education Accreditation (CNEA). (2021). *Accreditation Standards for Nursing Education Programs.* Washington, DC: NLN CNEA.

providers to "recognize and respond to the broader social, political, and economic structures that influence health and health care" (Davis & O'Brien, 2020, p. S59). Nurses and other health care providers engaged in structurally competent care also commit to the ongoing process of learning, self-reflection, collaboration, and advocacy in efforts to combat the multifaceted social and structural determinants of health inequities (Davis & O'Brien, 2020; Metzl & Hansen, 2014).

EDUCATIONAL STRATEGIES FOR SOCIAL AND STRUCTURAL DETERMINANTS OF HEALTH CURRICULUM

To effectively address SSDH in health care education, educational strategies that foster a comprehensive understanding of the complex interplay between social and structural determinants and health outcomes are needed. Such strategies must also emphasize the importance of addressing SSDH in clinical practice, research, and the role of health care practitioners in advocating for policy changes that promote health equity. Various educational strategies, including didactic lectures, case studies, simulations, and experiential learning activities, have been developed to address SSDH in health care education. These strategies can be tailored to meet the needs of diverse learners, including those from underrepresented backgrounds. See Table 1.2.

TABLE 1.2

Educational Strategies and Examples

Classroom Strategies	Examples
Discussions Deepen students' understanding by promoting critical thinking and active participation. Unlike passive methods, discussions enhance knowledge retention by encouraging students to articulate and debate concepts. Immediate feedback during discussions allows educators to promptly address misconceptions. Moreover, discussions foster a sense of community, encouraging self-reflection and open-mindedness.	Explore the social and structural determinants of Black infant mortality, including racism, and the potential role of epigenetic factors in this complex picture. Identify and justify two ethical principles that could be used to understand or reduce racism as an SSDH.
	Reflect on cultural arrogance or insensitivity in a health-related setting and the impact that cultural humility or structural competency training can have on preventing it. Explain a personal experience where cultural sensitivity, cultural humility, or knowledge of structural barriers was lacking in a health-related setting and how cultural humility or structural competency training could have prevented the occurrence.
	Describe three upstream factors (SSDH) associated with a selected health topic, explain how they might be measured, and specify which component of the Healthy People 2030 SSDH framework (ODPHP, n.d.) each factor addresses.

TABLE 1.2

Educational Strategies and Examples (*Continued*)

Classroom Strategies	Examples
Case Studies Immerse students in real-world scenarios and bridge theory with application. They foster critical thinking, prompting students to evaluate and synthesize information. Unlike traditional methods that emphasize memorization, case studies drive deeper comprehension and active participation. They provide an interdisciplinary learning experience, challenging students to draw connections across subjects. By presenting real-world dilemmas, case studies enhance decision-making skills and promote group collaboration, refining communication and teamwork. They also diversify assessment methods, catering to different learning styles. Importantly, case studies boost engagement, making learning relatable, and cultivate empathy by exposing students to diverse perspectives. Moreover, they prepare learners for real-life professional challenges that they may encounter in their careers.	Review case studies on the Millions Saved website (Center for Global Development, 2015). Describe the case study and why it is significant from a health care perspective. On the basis of the case study, explain the importance of customizing projects to meet local needs, evaluate whether the project demonstrates involvement of community members to advance health equity, and explain how methods used in the case study might be adapted to a different community or context. Navigate to the NLN (2022) ACE Pediatric Case Mia Jones. Have students discuss how the SSDH are affecting the client and identify interventions that can be implemented at the individual, family, and community level to minimize the effects of SSDH on this child and family.
Assignments Assignments offer a range of benefits in helping students develop essential knowledge, skills, and attributes needed for future careers. They assist the learner in critical thinking and application of knowledge, facilitate time management and research proficiency, and offer an opportunity for feedback from faculty for professional growth. Group assignments also promote teamwork, communication, and collaboration skills.	Research a major health problem that concerns a historically excluded or underrepresented population, the indicators of morbidity and mortality associated with the health problem, and how structural racism, urbanization, and poverty contribute to the problem. Create a narrated PowerPoint presentation on the relationship between water or food and health problems. Explain three SSDH related to the health problem, analyze how they are impacted by climate change, and propose a resolution to the problem. Write a paper on the role of health equity in the global distribution of disease and the importance of cultural humility and inclusion in public health research and planning. Propose at least two strategies to promote inclusion and equity within a public health program and system used in the region you selected. Assess the contributing factors (SSDH) to a health problem using a systems approach. Develop a conceptual framework with 6 to 10 connections between contributing factors, analyze how the ethical value of interdependence contributes to the system, and propose how organizations can collaborate to address SSDH. As part of a several-part project on community health assessment, explain what is known about a health issue of your choice, and provide recent local, state, and/or national sociodemographic, morbidity, and mortality data. Identify and describe one major contributing factor (SSDH) related to your health issue and recommend a meaningful gap that your community health assessment could address.

(*continued*)

TABLE 1.2

Educational Strategies and Examples (*Continued*)

Classroom Strategies	Examples
Concept Mapping Concept mapping is a visual teaching and learning strategy that helps the learner organize knowledge and ideas in an interconnected manner. Typically, concept maps consist of nodes (representing concepts) and lines or arrows (representing relationships) connecting these nodes. This strategy offers the benefits of promoting knowledge organization, critical thinking, memory enhancement, planning and decision-making, and collaboration.	Create a concept map in which the central node is labeled "Social and Structural Determinants of Health." From there, connect the various subnodes representing the different determinants, and outline how it can impact health outcomes. For example, when discussing "Access to Health Care," you might explain how limited access in rural areas can lead to inequities in health outcomes. Use arrows or lines to show how these factors are interconnected and influence each other.
	Pose this (or a similar simple, yet real-world clinical scenario) to learners: "A 16-year-old patient who lists her pronouns as she, her, and hers was recently diagnosed with type 2 diabetes." In phase one of the learning activity, ask learners to develop a concept map that outlines the patient's immediate and long-term care needs and education. In phase two, ask learners to examine how each domain of SSDH might impact this patient's health outcomes if they were living in a rural area, a suburban area, or a metropolitan area.

Clinical Strategies	Examples
Community-Based Partnerships Community-Based Partnerships (CBP) occur between academic institutions and community-based organizations (CBO) that are already providing services that address social determinants of health. Often CBOs have multiple partners within their network that specialize in different areas such as housing, food access, etc., to extend their reach and provide wraparound services to clients. Students in health professions programs can volunteer or engage in internships, field or clinical experiences to extend their learning about SSDH and address these at the community level. Students learn how to collaborate with CBOs, identify resources, and can contribute meaningfully to the work CBOs are doing to address SSDH.	Partner with a local fire department to receive referrals for non-urgent 911 calls that are due to health care and other access difficulties (McKinley Yoder & Pesch, 2020). Faculty and student teams can meet with clients over several weeks as care coordinators to address issues such as frequent falls, unsafe housing, accessing health care, or alcohol use disorder. Students have authentic learning experiences, including care coordination, interdisciplinary collaboration, identifying and accessing resources, and therapeutic communication. This also gives learners the opportunity to deeply understand the intersecting barriers to health that many people experience. Ask students to maintain documentation of their visits, strategies attempted, and evaluation, and then report this back to the fire department.
	Create a partnership with an organization that performs outreach to houseless populations. Often CBOs welcome short-term volunteers. Have students participate as a short-term volunteer, engage at least one client in a conversation, then reflect on how the experience challenged their preconceived ideas about people who are without housing.

TABLE 1.2

Educational Strategies and Examples (*Continued*)

Clinical Strategies	Examples
Clinical Experiences Health professions programs have clinical or field experiences as part of the curriculum. These experiences can take place in many different settings, including acute care, global, and community-based settings. Clinical experiences provide students with the opportunity to practice didactic and laboratory learning with individuals needing care under the supervision of licensed health care professionals.	As part of students' acute care clinical practicum, have students review the "Guide to Social Needs Screening" from the American Academy of Family Physicians (2023). Students should ask their patients each of the questions to identify SSDH that may affect the patient's ability to carry out the treatment plan, especially upon discharge. Then they can seek help for the client, provide resources, and alert the care team about potential barriers.
	In primary care settings, identify clients who are having difficulty following the prescribed treatment plan. Partner student pairs with the client as patient navigators to support clients overcoming barriers to treatment, such as poverty leading to inability to afford medications or unstable housing, limiting a client's ability to perform dressing changes for chronic leg ulcers. Clinical debriefings may include a discussion of upstream barriers.

Simulation-Based Strategies	Examples
Technology-Driven Simulations Virtual reality (VR) and digital (computer) simulations offer a dynamic approach to teaching SSDH, facilitating hands-on, immersive experiences that enhance retention and understanding. Conducted in a safe, controlled environment, simulations allow learners to explore diverse scenarios, fostering empathy and cultural competence. They promote skill development, from critical thinking to communication, and encourage interprofessional collaboration. With the added advantage of immediate feedback, learners can swiftly reflect on and improve their approaches. Furthermore, simulations resonate with real-world relevance, preparing health care professionals for practical challenges. Their adaptability ensures content remains current, reflecting evolving best practices and research.	Watch VR videos on resources in impoverished rural areas, then select one population impacted by structural barriers. Explain SSDH from the perspective of one of four main frameworks (WHO, Healthy People 2030, County Health Rankings, Kaiser Family Foundation) and evaluate how SSDH can guide surveillance data collection for the population selected.
	Use VR to transport nurses to a low-income neighborhood, allowing them to experience firsthand the structural barriers and challenges residents face in everyday life and in accessing health care.
	Create computer-based scenarios where health care professionals navigate patient stories, making decisions based on SSDH. Feedback can be provided in real-time, guiding learning.
Real-Life Interactions and Encounters Simulation with standardized patients, simulated home visits and skills labs are important modalities to help students practice skills, gain confidence in their role, and make mistakes in safe environments where they can learn without harming a patient. High-fidelity simulation using standardized patients creates an authentic experience allowing the student to learn to care for a patient with a low-occurrence, high-risk health problem such as cardiac arrest, placenta previa, or a manic episode which they would not necessarily encounter in clinical experiences.	Actors portray patients with diverse SSDH backgrounds in controlled settings with debriefing.
	Set up realistic home environments representing various socioeconomic backgrounds. This allows professionals to assess living conditions and understand how they impact health.
	Create mock clinical settings where professionals can practice skills like interviewing patients about SSDH or connecting patients with community resources.

(*continued*)

TABLE 1.2

Educational Strategies and Examples (*Continued*)

Simulation-Based Strategies	Examples
Group Activities and Collaborative Learning Role playing, tabletop scenarios, and interactive workshops allow students to develop team-based skills, engage in knowledge transfer, and practice communication skills that they can apply in practice.	Nurses and professionals switch roles with patients, experiencing health care scenarios from the patient's perspective, helping them understand barriers individuals might face due to SSDH.
	Use case studies and board game-style simulations to navigate complex patient scenarios, making decisions based on presented SSDH.
	Incorporate multimedia, storytelling, and group activities focused on specific determinants like housing, transportation, or nutrition.

Case Study: Walden University PhD in Public Health

Walden University's PhD in Public Health program was upgraded in 2021 to incorporate SSDH as a cross-cutting theme across all courses. The course of study was consciously structured to begin with fundamental concepts of SSDH—its terminology and definitions—and progress into more complex applications to real-world scenarios through an exploration of theory, ethics, measurement, research methods, and case studies.

The curriculum was subjected to a mixed methods evaluation in 2023 that demonstrated positive outcomes in both quantitative metrics and qualitative feedback, highlighting its effectiveness in enhancing student understanding and engagement. Course data, including pass rates and the analysis of specific learning artifacts, underlined the students' thorough grasp of the SSDH framework and its relevance to the field. A striking outcome was their substantial contribution to SSDH literature, with half of them focusing their research endeavors on this pivotal area. Qualitative feedback reinforced this data, with students expressing gratitude for the holistic approach to SSDH, which significantly shaped their viewpoints and analytical thinking.

A salient feature of the curriculum's success was its scaffolded design. This systematic layering of SSDH concepts ensured continuous reinforcement, enabling students to intertwine their understanding across courses. Even those with prior SSDH knowledge found their foundations enriched and broadened, underscoring the program's comprehensive nature. The aim was clear: to mold the next cadre of public health professionals, primed to combat health inequities and pave the way for a more equitable society.

STRATEGIES TO EVALUATE SOCIAL AND STRUCTURAL DETERMINANTS OF HEALTH CURRICULUM

Evaluating the integration and effectiveness of SSDH in academic curricula requires a comprehensive and multifaceted approach, combining both quantitative metrics and qualitative insights. By leveraging institutional data, analyzing student outputs, conducting in-depth interviews, and directly assessing course content, academic institutions can gain a robust understanding of the effectiveness and impact of their SSDH curriculum. This holistic approach ensures that the curriculum not only imparts knowledge but also equips students to apply SSDH principles in their future professional endeavors. The following strategies can be employed to assess SSDH curriculum comprehensively.

Adopt a Mixed Methods Research Design

Using a concurrent mixed methods research design to evaluate SSDH curriculum ensures that both quantitative and qualitative data are gathered simultaneously. This approach provides a more rounded understanding of the curriculum's effectiveness, impact, and areas for improvement, capturing both statistical outcomes and experiential narratives. Quantitative data may be collected to provide insights into curriculum effectiveness, student performance, and outcomes. Examples may include pre-/post-assessment scores, skills proficiency tests, standardized tests, attendance, participation, and completion rates, as well as survey data to gather student perceptions, confidence, and satisfaction with learning. Comparative data can also be used to explore curriculum impact.

Qualitative data may be gathered to offer in-depth insights into students' perceptions, experiences, and attitudes, including unexpected outcomes that might not be evident through quantitative measures alone. Examples may include individual or focus group interviews, narrative and thematic analysis, as well as content analysis of students' reflective journals or assignments. Observations and field notes, peer feedback, and other forms of anecdotal evidence can also provide valuable qualitative insights. By integrating quantitative measures with qualitative perspectives, educators gather a comprehensive dataset that guides curriculum improvement and aligns more effectively with the needs of both learners and communities.

Leverage Institutional Data

A primary source of quantitative data should be institutional records. Institutions can analyze grades recorded over specific terms to assess students' performance on SSDH-related artifacts from different courses. Key metrics to consider include pass rates, distribution of performance ratings, course completion rates, and evaluations, and the perceived difficulty level of various learning artifacts.

Assess Capstone Content

A robust indicator of a curriculum's influence on students' research endeavors is the thematic content of their capstone projects, theses, and dissertations. By examining titles, abstracts, and keywords of capstone documents, institutions can gauge the prominence of SSDH-focused research. Additionally, analyzing the theoretical frameworks employed, such as the socioecological model or ecosocial theory, provides insights into the depth and breadth of SSDH understanding imparted by the curriculum.

Conduct Qualitative Interviews

Direct feedback from students offers invaluable qualitative insights. By interviewing a diverse cohort of students, institutions can capture a range of experiences and perspectives. Using a semi-structured interview guide ensures consistency, while allowing space for students' unique narratives. Interviews can delve into students' perceptions of the SSDH curriculum, its real-world relevance, its challenges, and its impact on their academic and professional trajectories. Qualitative interviews can also function as a form of verbal examination, prompting students to articulate their definitions and understanding of SSDH and verify the depth of their comprehension.

Implement Rigorous Qualitative Analysis

After conducting interviews, a systematic approach to data analysis is crucial. Adopting strategies like those recommended by Creswell and Creswell (2023) ensures that the data are organized, relevant themes are identified, and meaningful narratives emerge. Key steps include employing content analysis and coding processes to segment and categorize data, generating descriptive summaries of settings and participants, and identifying and interpreting major themes.

Review Course Content and Structure

Beyond student feedback and performance metrics, a direct evaluation of the curriculum content is essential. This qualitative evaluation assesses the overall structure, format, and content depth of courses integrating SSDH. Key areas of focus include the completeness of SSDH topics covered, the depth of exploration, and the quality of instructional materials.

With institutional support, faculty teaching in online or blended courses can achieve course certification through Quality Matters (QM, 2023) or earn a QM Teaching Online Certificate. QM-certified courses undergo a rigorous peer-review process that objectively assesses various factors influencing the quality of the learner's experience in online or blended learning. These factors encompass course design, delivery, and content; institutional infrastructure; the learning management system; and the readiness of both faculty and learners (QM, 2023). Faculty interested in obtaining a Teaching Online Certificate from QM participate in a series of seven workshops that focus on different competencies that support online and blended delivery. This acknowledges that faculty play a pivotal role in both the design and delivery of courses. For educators seeking to incorporate SSDH concepts into their course designs and structures, guidance in quality assurance practices within higher education can be particularly beneficial. This approach ensures that SSDH-related content is seamlessly integrated while upholding established standards of excellence in course delivery and learner engagement.

CONCLUSION AND CALL TO ACTION

The integration of SSDH into health professions curricula goes beyond being a mere pedagogical decision; it represents a profound commitment to nurturing knowledgeable and compassionate professionals who are well equipped to advocate for health equity. Through the implementation of thoughtful strategies that prioritize student-centered learning, educational institutions possess the capacity to initiate a ripple effect that transforms academic insights into tangible societal changes. Institutions aiming to

TABLE 1.3

Strategies for Integrating SSDH into Curricula

Strategy	Description
Scaffolded learning	Begin with the basics and evolve to intricate layers of SSDH, ensuring students acquire a nuanced, phased understanding.
Cross-course integration	Instead of confining SSDH to one course, weave its principles across the program to underscore its universal relevance.
Diverse lenses	Equip students to view SSDH from varied angles—theory, ethics, research, and practical applications—enriching their comprehension.
Data-centric evaluation	Regularly gauge the curriculum's impact using both quantitative (pass rates, research contributions) and qualitative (student feedback) metrics.
Engaging pedagogy	Enliven the learning process with interactive methods, real-world examples, and immersive projects, making SSDH tangible and memorable.
Stay updated	Incorporate the latest SSDH research and findings to keep the curriculum fresh, relevant, and in sync with public health developments.
Practical emphasis	Highlight SSDH's real-world implications. Encourage students to translate their academic insights into actionable community health initiatives.
Leverage existing knowledge	Recognize students' prior SSDH exposure and craft the curriculum to amplify and expand their existing insights.
Faculty empowerment	Invest in faculty development, ensuring they are adept at delivering SSDH concepts engagingly and effectively.
Collaborative synergy	Promote interdisciplinary collaborations, marrying academic rigor with field expertise for a comprehensive SSDH educational experience.

seamlessly integrate SSDH into their curricula can consider the strategies presented in Table 1.3.

By conscientiously incorporating SSDH concepts into the curriculum, institutions empower their students to comprehend the multifaceted factors that influence health inequities. This comprehensive understanding serves as a cornerstone for future health care practitioners, enabling them to address the root causes of health inequities and contribute meaningfully to the well-being of individuals and communities. This commitment to SSDH education cultivates a sense of social responsibility among students. As they engage with the curriculum and gain insights into the impact of social and economic factors on health outcomes, they become advocates for change, committed to dismantling barriers to equitable health care access. This not only enriches their academic journey, but also equips them with the empathy and insight necessary to drive positive shifts in health care policies, practices, and public awareness.

Ultimately, the integration of SSDH into health professions curricula represents a transformative investment in the future of health care. By nurturing professionals who possess a comprehensive understanding of health determinants and their far-reaching implications, institutions shape leaders who are not only adept in their fields but are also dedicated to forging a more equitable and just health care landscape. This commitment transcends the classroom, creating a lasting impact that resonates throughout society and contributes to meaningful change.

Challenging Thoughts to Consider

1. How would a nurse or other health profession practitioners determine and examine the critical essentials of SSDH focused within their community as factors shaping the health outcomes of individuals versus communities?

2. Identify crucial strategies one can use to develop and transform a revised role for nurses and other health profession practitioners to better engage in meeting the diverse needs of their patients and communities.

3. What barriers to opportunities must one be aware of during design and implementation of SSDH into the curriculum to educate students as future practitioners and for faculty in the effective teaching of a strategic framework of SSDH in practice, implementation, and evaluation?

References

American Academy of Family Physicians (AAFP). (2023). *The EveryONE project: Assessment and action*. https://www.aafp.org/family-physician/patient-care/the-everyone-project/toolkit/assessment.html

Center for Global Development. (2015). *Millions Saved.* http://millionssaved.cgdev.org/

Creswell, J. W., & Creswell, J. D. (2023). *Research design: Qualitative, quantitative, and mixed methods approaches* (6th ed.). Sage.

Davis, S., & O'Brien, A. M. (2020). Let's talk about racism: strategies for building structural competency in nursing. *Academic Medicine, 95*(12), S58–S65. https://doi.org/10.1097/ACM.0000000000003688

Decker, R., Wagner, R., & Scholz, S. W. (2005). An internet-based approach to environmental scanning in marketing planning. *Marketing Intelligence & Planning, 23*(2), 189–199.

Fullan, M. (Ed.). (2005). *Fundamental change: International handbook of educational change.* Springer.

Hargreaves, A., & Fink, D. (2006). *Sustainable leadership*. Jossey-Bass.

Hyun, E. (2009). A study of US Academic Deans' involvement in college students' academic success. *International Studies in Educational Administration, 37*(2), 890110.

Lachiver, G., & Tardif, J. (2002). Fostering and managing curriculum change and innovation. *Proceedings Frontiers in Education Conference, 2*, F2–F7.

Layman, E., Bamberg, R., Campbell, C., & Wark, E. (2010). Environmental scanning: Allied health leaders' selection of strategic information. *Journal of Allied Health, 39*(1), 11–19.

Lemay, J., & Moreau, P. (2020). Managing a curriculum innovation process. *Pharmacy, 8*(3), 153. https://doi.org/10.3390/pharmacy8030153

Marijolovic, K. (2023). *How anti-DEI bills have already changed higher ed. The Chronicle of Higher Education.* https://www.chronicle.com/article/how-anti-dei-bills-have-already-changed-higher-ed

McKinley Yoder, C., & Pesch, M. S. (2020). An academic-fire department partnership to address social determinants of health. *Journal of Nursing Education, 59*(1), 34–37. https://doi.org/10.3928/01484834-20191223-08

Metzl, J. M., & Hansen, H. (2014). Structural competency: theorizing a new medical engagement with stigma and inequality. *Social Science & Medicine, 103*, 126–133. https://doi.org/10.1016/j.socscimed.2013.06.032

Myers, W. R. (2006). Essay: academic program assessment and the academic dean. In *ATS folio: master of divinity curriculum revision* (pp. 33–40). Association of Theological Schools.

National Academies of Sciences [NAS], formerly the Institute of Medicine [IOM]. (2003). *Health professions education: A bridge to quality.* National Academies Press. http://www.nap.edu/catalog/10681.html

National Academies of Sciences, Engineering, and Medicine (NASEM). (2016). Framing the dialogue on race and ethnicity to advance health equity: Proceedings of a Workshop (D.Thompson, Ed.). National Academies Press. https://www.nap.edu/catalog/23576

National Association of Diversity Officers in Higher Education (NADOHE). (2023, June 29). *Statement on the SCOTUS decisions on race-conscious admissions practices.* https://www.nadohe.org/statements/statement-scotus-race-conscious-admissions

National League for Nursing (NLN). (2023). *NLN urges nursing programs to value student diversity in the interest of public health.* NLN. https://www.nln.org/detail-pages/news/2023/07/06/nln-urges-nursing-programs-to-value-student-diversity-in-the-interest-of-public-health

National League for Nursing (NLN). (2022). *Advancing care excellence pediatrics: Mia Jones.* NLN. https://www.nln.org/education/teaching-resources/professional-development-programsteaching-resourcesace-all/acep/ace-p-unfolding-cases/mia-jones-5556c65c-7836-6c70-9642-ff00005f0421

National League for Nursing (NLN). Commission for Nursing Education Accreditation (CNEA). (2021, October). *Accreditation standards for nursing education programs.* NLN. https://irp.cdn-website.com/cc12ee87/files/uploaded/CNEA%20Standards%20October%202021-4b271cb2.pdf

National League for Nursing (NLN). (2019). *A vision for integration of the social determinants of health into nursing education curricula: A living document from the National League for Nursing.* NLN. http://www.nln.org/docs/default-source/default-documentlibrary/social-determinants-of-health.pdf?sfvrsn=2

Office of Disease Prevention and Health Promotion. (n.d.). Healthy People 2030. U.S. Department of Health and Human Services. https://health.gov/healthypeople

Oliver, S. L., & Hyun, E. (2011). Comprehensive curriculum reform in higher education: Collaborative engagement of faculty and administrators. *Journal of Case Studies in Education, 2*, 1–20. https://files.eric.ed.gov/fulltext/EJ1057195.pdf

Quality Matters (QM). (2023). *Quality matters overview.* https://www.qualitymatters.org/

Rudhumbu, N. (2015). Enablers of and barriers to successful curriculum in higher education: a literature review. *International Journal of Education Learning and Development, 3*(1), 12–26.

Suh, W. S., Key, S. K., & Munchus, G. (2004). Scanning behavior and strategic uncertainty. *Management Decision, 42*(8), 1001–1016.

Veltri, L. M. (2020). Forces and issues influencing curriculum development. In D. M. Billings & J. A. Halstead (Eds.), *Teaching in nursing: a guide for faculty* (6th ed., pp. 84–102). Elsevier.

World Health Organization Commission on Social Determinants of Health. (2008). *Closing the gap in a generation: health equity through action on the social determinants of health.* https://www.who.int/teams/social-determinants-of-health/equity-and-health/commission-on-social-determinants-of-health

Practice: Social and Structural Determinants of Health in Clinical Settings

Melissa Hinds, MSN, RN
Jannyse Tapp, DNP, FNP-BC

INTRODUCTION

Nurses and other health care providers aim to deliver high-quality care character-ized by safety, effectiveness, person-centeredness, timeliness, efficiency, and equity. Unequal health care quality for vulnerable populations can significantly influence health inequities and outcomes. It is essential to identify and implement strategies that help current and future health care professionals address social and structural determinants of health (SSDH) within both academic and practice settings. Although SSDH concepts have traditionally been taught primarily in community and public health courses, there's a growing recognition of the need to integrate these concepts into broader health care educational and clinical settings. This broader integration ensures that health care providers are well informed about SSDH, possess the neces-sary knowledge and tools to mitigate SSDH's impact on health outcomes, and can deliver more comprehensive care. This chapter discusses strategies aimed at creat-ing sustainable infrastructure and workflows for identifying, referring, and evaluating patients in need of social interventions. It also explores the integration of SSDH into nursing curricula and clinical practice, and the role of health care providers in advo-cating for social change to address health inequities.

Value and Alignwment

Reflecting on the National League for Nursing-Walden University Leadership Academy, we recognize that it has provided a yearlong journey for continuous learning and knowl-edge expansion. This experience has equipped us with new skills and tools to promote social change and advance health equity confidently and competently by incorporat-ing structural determinants into the SDH framework model (NASEM, 2021, p. 51). The opportunities to learn and grow in perspective and expertise have better prepared us to enhance our practices and that of others. This experience has also reinforced the importance of identifying and addressing SSDH.

Chapter Objectives

Upon completion of this chapter, the learner will be able to:

1. Learn strategies for incorporating SSDH within diverse educational and clinical settings.
2. Identify tools and resources to help the emerging workforce and providers in practice to reduce health inequalities.

INTEGRATING SOCIAL AND STRUCTURAL DETERMINANTS OF HEALTH IN PRACTICE: IT STARTS IN THE ACADEMIC SETTING

Medical care contributes to only 10 to 20 percent of modifiable factors impacting population health, while the remaining 80 to 90 percent is attributed to social determinants (County Health Rankings & Roadmaps, 2022). A 2019 Kaiser Permanente study found that nearly 70 percent of individuals faced at least one social determinant challenge at some point (Kaiser Permamemte, 2019). Consequently, assessing and managing SSDH are vital competencies for health care professionals. As emphasized in the 2019 National League for Nursing (NLN) Call for Action, "assessment of SSDH, along with a physical, cultural, and functional assessment of patients, families, and communities, is an essential competency" (NLN, 2019, p. 5). Integrating SSDH into health professions curricula through experiential learning in academic programs, clinical rotations, and various health care settings equips health care providers to address social needs and emerging roles in advancing health equity.

Social needs refer to the social and economic needs that individuals experience that affect their ability to maintain their health and well-being. The SSDH refer to how factors such as institutional racism, bias, and racism influence the distribution of money, power, and resources and impact the conditions in which people are born, grow, work, live, and age (NASEM, 2017; NASEM, 2021). In effect, SSDH causes inequities in social needs (Alderwick & Gottlieb, 2019). Addressing social needs is a crucial component of efforts to mitigate the impact of social determinants on health and promote overall well-being. To effectively identify and support patients with unmet social needs, it is essential to understand patient characteristics and the types of unmet social needs within diverse populations. It is important to emphasize that social needs depend on individual preferences and priorities. This highlights the essential role of person-centered care and shared decision-making (Alderwick & Gottlieb, 2019; Chepatis et al., 2021; Green & Zook, 2019). Social needs are social conditions that present the most challenges for individuals (Alderwick & Gottlieb, 2019; Chepatis et al., 2021; Green & Zook, 2019).

Education and training are crucial elements in integrating SSDH into practice. Even individuals, including providers, educators, and students, who recognized SSDH's significance may not routinely screen for them due to a lack of training or awareness of available resources for referrals. Additionally, some may feel uncomfortable or ill-prepared to broach sensitive topics like food access or income levels. Nevertheless, assessing SSDH issues can render care plans practical and feasible. Understanding how these factors influence health can facilitate the development and implementation of more effective health promotion programs and policies. Consequently, a greater emphasis on training and opportunities to practice assessment skills and interventions is needed for gaining insight into community health needs and delivering adequate care.

Preparation starts in the academic setting to ensure that students are ready for reducing inequities in practice by recognizing different patient needs and preferences. Screening for SSDH and screening for social needs should be part of the practicing health care professional's curriculum.

The exemplar in Table 2.1 describes the integration of an SSDH tool (the tool is shown in Table 2.2) into clinical documentation.

TABLE 2.1

Exemplar: Integration of an SSDH Tool into Clinical Documentation for MSN Specialty Students

Component	Description and Rationale
Introduction	Persistent health inequities across the United States result from social and structural determinants of health (SSDH), leading to inequities in morbidity and mortality among certain groups. These inequities disproportionately affect underrepresented populations, resulting in preventable differences in health and health care access that perpetuate inequities. Addressing these complex issues requires a collective cross-professional effort, with nurses playing a crucial role in mitigating SSDHs on health outcomes.
	Nurses must be prepared to address SSDH in practice by integrating SSDH education into nursing curricula (Thornton & Persaud, 2018). Equipping nurses with the knowledge to address SSDH in all patient populations, especially underrepresented ones, promotes equitable and quality health care. The aim is to prepare future nurse practitioners to provide equitable care that considers the influence of SSDH on individual patients.
	Institutional restructuring allows an opportunity to evaluate the integration of SSDH across all levels of education. Commonly, variations exist based on specialty population focus. To ensure consistent SSDH coverage at the master's level, concepts may be introduced into a Health Assessment course. This approach aligns with the need for consistent assessments and documentation (Bradywood et al., 2021). Their study revealed that the absence of formal tools for capturing social risk factors led to insufficient and inconsistent information, potentially harming patient outcomes. Thus, routine patient screening must be conducted adequately.
	Beyond didactic instruction, preparing students for effective SSDH practice required the development of an assessment tool for evaluating their application of SSDH concepts during clinical rotations. This tool aligns with specialty-specific clinical documentation guidelines, particularly the Subjective, Objective, Assessment and Plan (SOAP) note. It ensures students' incorporation of SSDH into patient care is assessed comprehensively, a crucial aspect of their readiness for practice. Notably, despite the well-documented impact of SSDH, primary care providers often lack a structured approach to addressing patients' nonmedical social needs in clinic settings (Page-Reeves et al., 2016).
	The tool's development aimed to dissolve historical silos among specialties, fostering a holistic health care approach that acknowledges SSDH's influence across patient populations. Consistent SSDH assessment in clinical experiences aims to heighten students' awareness of these determinants, enhancing their advocacy skills for addressing them. The goal is to empower future nurse practitioners to reduce health inequities and contribute to a more equitable and just health care system for all.

(continued)

TABLE 2.1

Exemplar: Integration of an SSDH Tool into Clinical Documentation for MSN Specialty Students (*Continued*)

Component	Description and Rationale
Why Is Screening Important?	Screening for SSDH in health care is crucial. It enables holistic patient care by considering socioeconomic status, education, housing, employment, and resource access. This comprehensive approach allows health care providers to offer personalized, effective care, considering patients' broader context and challenges (Anderman, 2018). Moreover, it addresses root causes of health issues, as many inequities and chronic conditions stem from social determinants. By providing resources to overcome these barriers, health care providers empower patients to manage their health, adhere to treatments, and improve well-being. Furthermore, screening for SSDH can curb health care costs. Unaddressed social determinants lead to increased health care utilization and costs. Patients with social challenges often visit emergency rooms and have more hospitalizations due to poorly managed conditions. Addressing these determinants can potentially cut health care expenses (Anderman, 2018). Lastly, screening aligns with the paramount goal of promoting health equity. It enables providers to address inequities in underrepresented populations, working toward a more just and equitable health care system.
SWOT Analysis: Vanderbilt University School of Nursing	After conducting a SWOT (Strengths, Weaknesses, Opportunities, Threats) analysis, key findings emerged. Vanderbilt University School of Nursing (VUSN) exhibited strengths, firmly committed to equity, diversity, and inclusion, which includes integrating SSDH into the curriculum. Additionally, previous attempts at introducing SSDH content and administrative buy-in, coupled with ongoing restructuring in the Advanced Health Assessment course, provided an ideal environment for project development.
	Nonetheless, weaknesses needed attention, such as inconsistent content delivery among specialties, specialty silos, and divergent clinical documentation guidelines. These challenges, viewed as opportunities due to varied patient populations and underserved clinical sites, enhanced the project. Potential threats included specialty resistance to changing documentation practices and preceptor unfamiliarity with SSDH's clinical significance.
	Despite challenges, the SWOT analysis reaffirmed the project's urgency and feasibility. Leveraging VUSN's commitment to equity, diversity, and inclusion and addressing weaknesses through interspecialty collaboration promised a cohesive approach. Diverse patient populations and clinical settings provided unique implementation opportunities. To mitigate threats, open communication and education were vital for fostering understanding among stakeholders.
	This SWOT analysis recognized the project's potential to impact nursing education and clinical practice by addressing SSDH, promoting better health care outcomes and equity.

TABLE 2.1

Exemplar: Integration of an SSDH Tool into Clinical Documentation for MSN Specialty Students (Continued)

Component	Description and Rationale
Available Screening Tools	Various screening tools are available for health care providers to identify SSDH in patients. The selection of a screening tool should consider the specific social determinants under assessment and the health care context. However, beyond identification, health care providers must also ensure they have the necessary resources and support systems in place to address these needs effectively. Here are commonly used instruments in health care settings. ***PRAPARE (Protocol for Responding to and Assessing Patients' Assets, Risks, and Experiences)*** PRAPARE is a versatile and widely recognized screening tool. It comprehensively evaluates factors beyond medical conditions, including housing stability, food security, income, education, and employment status. Initially used in community health centers, PRAPARE is now expanding to hospitals, health systems, and health plans (Weir et al., 2020). ***The Health Leads Social Needs Screening Toolkit*** The Health Leads Social Needs Screening Toolkit offers a range of screening tools for different social determinants, including housing, food, utilities, transportation, childcare, employment, legal assistance, safety, and mental health challenges like social isolation (The Health Leads Screening Toolkit, 2018). https://healthleadsusa.org/communications-center/resources/the-health-leads-screening-toolkit/ ***Accountable Health Communities Health-Related Social Needs Screening Tool*** The Accountable Health Communities Health-Related Social Needs Screening Tool, part of the CMS' Accountable Health Communities Model, evaluates five key domains: housing instability, food insecurity, transportation needs, utility needs, and interpersonal safety (Billioux et al., 2017). ***The Hunger Vital Sign*** The Hunger Vital Sign is a validated two-question screening tool to identify patient food insecurity. It is a reliable indicator of household food insecurity (Gattu et al., 2019). ***Core 5 SSDH Screening Checklist*** The Core 5 SSDH screening checklist examines patients' housing instability, food insecurity, utility needs, transportation barriers, and interpersonal violence (Bechtel et al., 2022). **Adapted SSDH Screening Tool** The developed SSDH screening tool, derived from validated instruments, aims to provide versatility across various specialties and clinical settings, catering to different age groups, from pediatrics to adults. To streamline use, it excludes questions already available in the patient's chart, such as race/ethnicity, language, and alcohol and tobacco use, as these are typically recorded in electronic medical records or intake questionnaires. However, students are encouraged to inquire about these topics when necessary, ensuring accurate information. The remaining questions in the tool should be consistently asked by Advanced Practice Registered Nursing (APRN) students during clinical encounters. This data should be integrated into clinical documentation and decision-making. It is recommended that specialty programs incorporate this tool into their clinical documentation process and adapt grading rubrics accordingly. Every student should proactively use the tool during patient encounters, incorporating SSDH data into treatment or referral plans. This patient-centered approach enhances holistic care and improves patient outcomes.

(continued)

TABLE 2.1

Exemplar: Integration of an SSDH Tool into Clinical Documentation for MSN Specialty Students (*Continued*)

Component	Description and Rationale
Evaluation Plan	An extensive evaluation plan will be implemented to assess the impact and effectiveness of the Advanced Health Assessment content template and the SSDH assessment tool in clinical practice. This plan will encompass survey-based feedback and rubric-guided evaluations.
	A survey, adapted from Muirhead et al. (2022), will gauge students' perceptions of their SSDH knowledge, skills, and confidence. Administered at the program's start and completion, this longitudinal approach tracks improvements in students' SSDH competency throughout their studies. Qualitative feedback from the survey will offer insights into students' experiences and challenges, integrating SSDH into clinical practice.
	To evaluate the SSDH tool in clinical documentation, faculty will integrate SSDH criteria into the clinical documentation rubric. This will assess students' incorporation of SSDH into patient assessments and its impact on management plans. Specialties will collaborate to ensure consistency and fairness.
	Combining survey data and rubric-guided evaluations provide a comprehensive view of the content and tool's impact. This data-driven approach informs curriculum and tool enhancements, ultimately preparing students to address SSDH and deliver patient-centered care effectively.
Conclusion	Despite the availability of screening tools for clinical settings, a specific tool for academic clinical documentation was lacking. The resultant adapted tool is now a concise and comprehensive instrument designed for seamless integration across specialties (see Table 2.2). It is essential for student nurse practitioners to use this tool to assess and address SSDH competently. As nurse educators, we aim to equip students to become the next generation of health care providers who can effectively tackle health inequities.

TABLE 2.2

SSDH Clinical Documentation Tool

Domain	Recommended Question	Published Screening Tool	Student Considerations	Student Interventions
Education	What is your highest level of education?	PRAPARE	Literacy, health literacy, written or verbal instructions, patient education	Tailor patient education to literacy/health literacy level. Provide written or verbal instructions based on patient need

TABLE 2.2

SSDH Clinical Documentation Tool (*Continued*)

Domain	Recommended Question	Published Screening Tool	Student Considerations	Student Interventions
Employment	Are you currently employed?	PRAPARE	Cost of treatment plan, impact of missed days of work	Manage multiple complaints during visit (if possible) to avoid missed days, consider resources to reduce cost burden to patient (Good prescription, insurance formulary, patient assistance programs)
Food Security	Do you or your family worry about getting enough food to eat?	PRAPARE, Core 5	Patient education, impact of poor nutrition	Referral to social services, local religious organizations, local food pantries
Housing	Do you have housing? Are you homeless? (shelter, friend or family house, hotel)	PRAPARE, Core 5	Patient safety	Referral to social services
Transportation	Is transportation a concern? Has a lack of transportation prevented you from attending work or medical appointments?	Core 5	Missed or late appointments	Consolidate return visits, refer to social services for transportation assistance
Exposure to Violence	Do you feel safe in your home or neighborhood? Are you worried that someone may hurt you or your family?	Core 5	Safe to navigate neighborhood	Research community resources (community centers, YMCA) Refer for IPV intervention services
Financial hardship	How hard is it for you to pay for daily necessities? Food, utilities, medication, transportation, child care, etc.?	PRAPARE, Core 5	Impacts of weather (extreme heat or cold), refrigeration for medication, as needed	Refer to social services

PRAPARE, Protocol for Responding to and Assessing Patients' Assets, Risks, and Experiences.

Strategies for Implementation and Integration of Social Determinants of Health in Clinical Practice

To address the changing landscape and needs of individuals, a fundamental shift from patient-centered to person-centered care in the health care system is crucial (NASEN, 2021). *Patient-centered care* revolves around individual interactions within health care, focusing on the patient. In contrast, *person-centered care* encompasses a broader understanding of individuals within their communities, considering their health, psychosocial needs, and community context. While patient-centered care aims for a functional life for the patient, person-centered care strives for a meaningful life. The goal is to create training tools and resources that enhance provider knowledge, offering practical suggestions and resources for addressing SSDH, and supplementing other person-centered competencies.

Understanding the difference between upstream and downstream SSDH is extremely important. Upstream social determinants are the root causes of health issues and health outcomes (Braveman & Gottlieb, 2014; NASEM, 2021). Downstream social determinants are factors that are temporarily and spatially close to health issues and health outcomes and are influenced by upstream factors (Braveman et al., 2011; Davis, 2022). Addressing downstream social needs, while necessary, does not address the underlying upstream systemic and structural issues that caused the downstream problem in the first place (Davis, 2022; NASEM, 2017 and Ray et al., 2023). Mental health professionals, for example, often deal with downstream effects of social determinants, but addressing upstream factors is vital for improved mental health outcomes (Shim & Compton, 2018). This approach can promote population-level mental health and prevention strategies. However, a significant challenge is that provider training typically focuses on diseases and mental health rather than on SSDH. Providers need to obtain more knowledge and competency in evaluating and addressing SSDH.

Systems and agencies working to advance the behavioral health care workforce must provide the highest quality and value in services and evidence-based treatments for recovery and wellness to service recipients and their families. As outlined in the exemplar in Table 2.3, a SWOT (Strengths, Weaknesses, Opportunities, Threats) analysis revealed challenges in collecting SSDH data, time constraints on providers, and varying infrastructure for capturing SSDH information statewide. The Center for Practice Innovations (CPI) works to advance the behavioral health care workforce's ability to deliver high-quality, evidence-based care and treatments for recovery (Center for Practice Innovations, 2024). This experience can benefit other settings in their quality improvement and training efforts.

To address the challenges identified in the SWOT analysis, better integration of the concept of SSDH into all new and previously created content within the training curriculum was needed. Effectively addressing SSDH and their associated needs requires interprofessional team members to comprehend each member's role, both direct and indirect, in the awareness, assistance, and advocacy activities. Team members should maintain their professional identity while understanding the knowledge, skills, and competencies of others. This improved integration of SSDH clarifies the "why" and "how" of interprofessional collaboration, which is essential to their work.

A primary goal of the CPI and the New York State (NYS) Office of Mental Health (OMH) is to build upon and expand diversity, equity, inclusion, and social justice-related initiatives already under way statewide New York State Office of Mental Health.

(n.d.) https://omh.ny.gov/. Given the complexity of the behavioral health system and the diversity of NYS's residents, securing buy-in from various stakeholders was crucial (Wark et al., 2022). The SWOT analysis led to the formulation of implementation and training redesign principles, including 1) reviewing SSDH; 2) exploring the impact of SSDH on care; 3) recognizing the roles of providers, the emerging workforce, and behavioral health organizations in reducing health inequity; 4) identifying practical recommendations for addressing SSDH in behavioral health care settings; and 5) providing references for existing community resources.

CPI has an interprofessional leadership group that actively participated in coordinating the content and overall module development. The NYS OMH, which serves dual roles in licensing and oversight, also has played a crucial role in the implementation and dissemination of this resource. The OMH facilitated the resource's adoption within the settings they operate, extended it to agencies under their licensing purview, and distributed it to contracted behavioral health, managed care organizations.

Developing a Training Plan

Improving the focus on SSDH within the training curricula of behavioral health organizations is most effectively achieved by ensuring that a diverse group of providers and staff from various racial and ethnic underrepresented backgrounds have equal access to training opportunities and resources (Wyse et al., 2020). Programs can seamlessly integrate SSDH throughout their training course curricula and offer the workforce readily available, easily accessible, and translatable education materials; technological tools; and community-based resources.

Ongoing Professional Development

The CPI functions as an intermediary organization and serves as one of the training institutes under the OMH, with the goal of increasing the competencies of the NYS's behavioral health workforce and facilitating the practical application of this training within agencies and organizations. By conducting these training activities within a not-for-profit context rather than the state system, CPI reduces barriers to accessing SSDH resources in settings beyond the OMH. This approach encourages cross-agency and cross-regional collaboration among staff.

CPI's leadership convenes biannually to review the current work plan, emerging areas of interest, and activities that involve local community partners. Regular stakeholder and provider community meetings provide a platform for all parties to address gaps in employee knowledge, identify additional training needs or technical assistance, and formulate data-driven recommendations. For example, each stakeholder group contributes to the dissemination and updates on how SSDH is assessed, tracked, and managed within their respective domains. CPI collects this information through its LMS, utilizing level 1 (reaction), level 2 (knowledge), and level 3 (behavior change) evaluations. The synthesized data inform the revision of existing content and the creation of new materials, as well as the identification of supplementary support measures.

For behavioral health professions, lifelong learning is often facilitated through continuing professional development and continuing education. Health professionals require

---

BOX 2.1

Overview of Project Structures

COMPONENTS: Design, create, test, and analyze an asynchronous module on SSDH

Phase I: Module Design and Development

> **Activity 1:** Create draft
> **Activity 2:** Share content with CPI leadership and OMH for review, edits, and approval
> **Activity 3:** Collaborate with the module developer to create a 30-45-minute online module
> **Activity 4:** Develop level 1, 2 and/or level 3 evaluations that will be attached to the module
> **Activity 5:** Submit content for continuing education units (CEU) approval
> **Activity 6:** Test and approve the final version of the module

Phase II: Module Dissemination

> **Activity 1:** Create and trigger a marketing campaign about the training module
> **Activity 2:** Add new resource announcement to the CPI website
> **Activity 3:** Coordinate provider network dissemination with OMH
> **Activity 4:** Conduct initial post-dissemination assessment

Phase III: Evaluation and Analysis of Resources

> **Activity 1:** Analyze user feedback data 30 days post-dissemination
> **Activity 2:** Produce reports of results
> **Activity 3:** Summarize module findings at 3-month/90-day follow-up

---

access to education that fosters critical thinking and offers transformative learning opportunities, from foundational education to ongoing professional development. Numerous opportunities exist for organizational leaders and staff to engage in learning experiences related to SSDH and health care. The redesigned training curriculum offers staff the chance to deepen their understanding of SSDH, community health needs, population health, patient engagement, and outcomes. These opportunities are provided through eLearning courses, webinars, and learning communities, benefiting around 27,000 individuals across New York. For example, one of the training components, the eLearning course *Foundations of the Social Determinants of Health*, aims to educate providers and evaluate their confidence and self-efficacy in addressing SSDH. Box 2.1 outlines the design, creation, testing, and analysis of an asynchronous module on SSDH.

Integrating interprofessional workplace learning into everyday practice is a means of providing busy health care providers with real-time education and interactions on how social, political, and economic conditions influence individual and population health. Professional development of the provider can enhance their confidence in identifying interventions and addressing the discomfort associated with screenings, promoting ongoing engagement and problem-solving. Using validated screening tools to screen patients can help overcome time constraints and alleviate staff-patient discomfort. Health systems or programs aiming to implement social needs and SSDH screening should carefully strategize to boost staff motivation and readiness for implementation. Developing clear methods and policies can enhance the staff-patient screening experience and evaluate their impact on reach and effectiveness (Counts, 2023).

Assessing Competencies Related to SSDH

When integrating SSDH into a behavioral health training curriculum, it is essential to acknowledge its current status and future direction (Alegría et al., 2018). Coordinating these themes across content and practice settings is complex, but the CPI plays a pivotal role in training dissemination. Through technical assistance, CPI has paved the way to raise awareness of SSDH and create a culture in which discussing SSDH is a natural part of the conversation. As health care programs and training settings respond to the increasing need for competency measurements related to SSDH, the work must cater to diverse programs and settings. While SSDH is integrated into our overall competency model, we are still in the process of developing and operationalizing specific SSDH skills, encompassing both "hard" and "soft" skill development. Our aim is to emphasize that identifying and addressing SSDH goes beyond a mere checkbox; it genuinely impacts communities and reduces barriers to mental health care through well-informed, policy-level decisions.

Developing competencies that foster interprofessional collaboration is an essential element of transformative learning for addressing SSDH and providing comprehensive training opportunities (Boss & Gulley, 2022). Nurses, psychiatrists, psychologists, social workers, peers, and other staff members collaborate to address patients' non-health needs, ultimately enhancing their overall health. Learners encompass a diverse group, including staff members, the emerging workforce, and community workers, who engage in service-learning experiences with various behavioral health settings (e.g., inpatient units, mental health clinics, and federally qualified health centers). These settings are increasingly incorporating the assessment and mitigation of SSDH into their program outcomes. Proficiency in SSDH is integral to service delivery and achieving program outcomes. SSDH-related content is evaluated across several domains, including critical thinking and analysis, management, and knowledge. For example, in the online course *Foundations of Social Determinants of Health,* learners begin by completing a pre-survey to establish their baseline knowledge. Throughout the course, they refine their understanding of SSDH through self-reflection, application exercises, and service-learning opportunities, leading to a comprehensive grasp of these critical concepts.

The curriculum seamlessly integrates an understanding of health inequities and the factors driving these inequities into our existing training programs, focusing on health-related social needs, bias, and systemic oppression. Learners begin by familiarizing themselves with key terminology and definitions related to the course content. They delve into the concept of good health, examining the multifaceted factors influencing an individual's well-being. The course explores health inequities, offering state or regional health disparity statistics to illuminate the extent of these inequities. Learners investigate the root causes behind these inequities, considering factors relevant to various populations, including immigrants, migrants, veterans, individuals experiencing homelessness, and others. The curriculum also delves into the upstream, midstream, and downstream factors of SSDH, while introducing the Social Needs Model. To apply their newfound knowledge, learners engage in case studies. Successful completion of the course culminates in a quiz and a post-course knowledge evaluation. This training equips internal and behavioral health staff across various settings to harness outcome data (Artiga & Hinton, 2018) effectively, enhancing our capacity to understand unmet needs and deliver optimal care.

As training requirements and staff development priorities continue to evolve, the integration of training platforms as a strategic tool enables organizations to create, implement, and assess new curricula, providing staff with adaptable skill sets for their practice. Engaging in this service-learning curriculum offers providers the opportunity to cultivate humility in their patient interactions while fostering a fresh perspective on the quality of care they can deliver. Furthermore, replicating this curriculum across various stakeholder groups enables multiple organizations to establish standardized approaches to address nonclinical SSDH, often extending beyond the reach of individual providers. See Table 2.3.

Transitioning from academia to clinical practice is a pivotal step in shaping health care professionals capable of delivering high-quality, person-centered care. As highlighted by the NLN in 2019, failing to intentionally integrate SSDH in clinical settings and training programs can have unintended consequences, contributing to unequal health care quality and perpetuating health inequities (NLN, 2019). The evolving landscape of health care education recognizes the imperative to extend the traditional focus on SSDH from community and public health courses to a broader integration across various nursing courses, health care disciplines, and clinical settings. This expansion ensures that health care providers possess the requisite knowledge and tools to address SSDH's impact on health outcomes, fostering a more comprehensive approach to patient care. By starting in the academic setting, we lay the groundwork for health care professionals to adeptly navigate the complexities of SSDH, thereby fostering a more equitable and effective health care system.

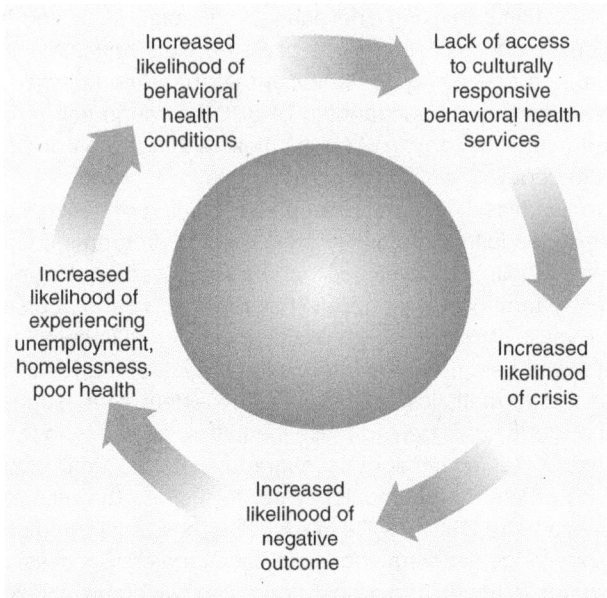

FIGURE 2.1 Community Intervention Opportunity Cycle.

TABLE 2.3

Exemplar: Clinical Setting: Foundations of Social Determinants of Health: Educating Providers and the Emerging Mental Health Workforce on the Social Determinants of Health

The Challenge or Opportunity	Explanation
Introduction	Social and structural determinants of health (SSDH) have a sweeping influence on health care, health policy, and public health. Neglecting SSDH perpetuates a cycle of health inequities and inequality. Factors that negatively impact SSDH include poor lifestyle choices and health behaviors, limited socioeconomic opportunities, sociocultural factors, such as values and education, plus restricted access to social and natural resources, coupled with living in unsafe environments with high violence rates and health risks.
	Practitioners encounter obstacles in addressing health equity and social determinants in routine care. The Root Cause Coalition (2020) revealed that 71% of primary care providers, 69% of nurse practitioners, and 76% of physician assistants needed more to discuss social risk factors during appointments. Another study found 63% of respondents required adequate resources and strategies to integrate clinical resources with community partners (Heath, 2020). Although awareness is growing that health improvement and equity entail broader approaches considering social, economic, justice, and environmental factors, there's a significant gap in addressing SSDH through behavioral health initiatives and policies. Thus, prioritizing behavioral health equity is crucial for addressing SSDH comprehensively.
	In New York State, about 30% reside upstate, while the majority live downstate, encompassing New York City, Long Island, and Hudson River counties (U.S. Census Bureau, 2023). Geographic location can expose individuals to varying environmental risks, chronically underresourced health care systems, and intergenerational historical trauma (McKnight-Eily et al., 2021). Beyond its physical impacts, SSDH also significantly affects mental health. Factors like unemployment, unstable employment, and working conditions are associated with increased psychological distress (Pevalin et al., 2017). Lower incomes and financial strain can lead to mental health issues, including self-harm, suicide attempts, and depression (Alegría et al., 2018).
	Discrimination, be it based on race, sexual orientation, occupation, or immigration status, consistently correlates with adverse mental health in the U.S. Community violence exposure in adolescence relates to higher depression, anxiety, and PTSD symptoms (Alegría et al., 2018). High local prison admission rates can increase the risk of major depressive or generalized anxiety disorder (Khan et al., 2017). On the positive side, strong familial bonds, social support, community belonging, and trust in others enhance mental health (Alegría et al., 2018). Perceived emotional support and support network size protect against common mental health disorders, personality dysfunction, and psychotic experiences (Alegría et al., 2018).
	Historically underrepresented communities disproportionally suffer from inadequate access to quality, culturally responsive behavioral health care, compounding mental health issues (Boss & Gulley, 2022). This perpetuates health inequities (see Figure 2.1). At each stage, there are opportunities for intervention and collaboration to address inequities and improve behavioral health services. Actions include upstream interventions, advocating for policies that address mental health's social determinants, and potentially reducing adverse childhood experiences, poverty income inequality, and improving education and employment opportunities for all (Shim & Compton, 2018).
	Addressing SSDH is possible and crucial for health systems. Enhancing provider education on tackling SSDH and promoting health equity across diverse populations is vital (Wark et al., 2022). This requires better preparing providers for diverse practice settings and populations. Governments, health systems, educators, and payers must leverage programmatic, policy, and funding opportunities to expedite these improvements uniformly and effectively (NASEM, 2021).

(*continued*)

TABLE 2.3

Exemplar: Clinical Setting: Foundations of Social Determinants of Health: Educating Providers and the Emerging Mental Health Workforce on the Social Determinants of Health (*Continued*)

The Challenge or Opportunity	Explanation
The Challenge	Behavioral health is integral to well-being, but the U.S. faces a mental health crisis. In 2020, 21.0% of adults had any mental illness, 5.6% had a serious mental illness (SMI), and 14.5% had a substance use disorder (SUD), with 6.7% having co-occurring disorders (SAMHSA, 2021). Poor mental health and substance misuse impact choices, living conditions, and opportunities (NIDA, 2022). Notably, the mortality difference between the general population and individuals with SMI or SUD face a 10- to 25-year mortality gap, with many avoidable deaths (de Mooij et al., 2019).
	Addressing social determinants is crucial for individuals with behavioral health conditions due to higher mortality rates and the complex interplay between mental health, substance use, physical health, and social factors (Artiga & Hinton, 2018). Interventions are often one-dimensional, focusing on specific domains (e.g., employment or housing). To address multiple social determinants effectively, providers need a comprehensive understanding of the full spectrum of SSDH (Root Cause Coalition, 2020). This multifaceted approach can mitigate systemic social inequalities and enhance patient support.
	The absence of SSDH in competency standards often necessitates ongoing learning for providers and students during their practice. This knowledge gap can affect the preparedness of the behavioral workforce to address inequities in health care. Focusing on upstream SSDH factors can prevent health issues rather than just treating them. Until SSDH training becomes a core competency, the proposed resource can bridge this knowledge and practice gap (Wark et al., 2022). Racial, ethnic, and socioeconomic inequities significantly impact mortality rates and life expectancy. Unlike the other determinants, individuals can't control their birth surroundings, race, or socioeconomic status (SES). These are SDH because different SES and racial groups exhibit different health outcomes and behaviors. For example, lower SES is associated with increased smoking, less physical activity, poorer diets, higher disability rates, and shorter lifespans (Deferio et al., 2019).
	Providers play a pivotal role in addressing social and structural determinants of health, which significantly influence overall wellness, with nearly 80% of it being nonclinical. To ensure holistic care that considers all health determinants, providers must continuously learn and increase their knowledge regarding SSDH and health inequities' impact on outcomes. Understanding and addressing SSDH is essential for delivering high-quality care, improving SSDH and health outcomes, and dismantling social and policy barriers. The Center for Practice Innovations (CPI) facilitates provider support in addressing SSDH and social needs through clinical policy and practice interventions. Here, we detail how CPI's resource equips providers with both knowledge and practical tools for this purpose.

TABLE 2.3

Exemplar: Clinical Setting: Foundations of Social Determinants of Health: Educating Providers and the Emerging Mental Health Workforce on the Social Determinants of Health (*Continued*)

The Challenge or Opportunity	Explanation
The Opportunity	As we transition from traditional service delivery to community-based engagement, providers must be able to practice to the fullest scope of their education, training, and competencies. Continuous learning is essential for comprehending the impact of factors like SSDH and health inequities on outcomes. To facilitate this transition from theory to practice, this resource offers both knowledge and practical tools. Its aim is to empower providers to deliver higher-quality care, improve SSDH and health outcomes, and actively address social and policy barriers in their roles.
	The Center for Practice Innovations (CPI) is committed to promoting evidence-based practices (EBP) for individuals with behavioral health conditions and advancing integrated care. Serving as a bridge between research and practice, CPI facilitates capacity-building agencies and systems to ensure the sustainability of EBPs. CPI maintains a close working relationship with external entities like the Office of Mental Health (OMH), aiding in policy development, program guidance, licensing requirements, and provider education. Additionally, CPI assists community behavioral health providers in adapting to external influences through training, barrier removal strategies, and ongoing support during EBP implementation and sustainability efforts.
	CPI's Learning Management System (LMS) offers accessible and continuous staff development, technical assistance, and education to nonprofit behavioral health providers and students pursuing degrees in behavioral health care. The LMS provides access to high-quality, evidence-based training and best practices while enabling data collection for evaluation purposes (reaction, knowledge, and behavior levels). CPI further contributes to the OMH's mission of promoting EBPs statewide by offering continuing education (CE) credits to various health professionals in New York State, including physicians, psychologists, licensed counselors, social workers, nurses, and substance use counselors.
Assessing Training at the Center for Practice Innovations for the Integration of SSDH	Applying an informal SWOT (Strengths, Weaknesses, Opportunities, Threats) framework identified key considerations in utilizing SDH knowledge for health outcomes. Strengths include the LMS, accreditation capabilities for training, and an interprofessional user base. Weaknesses entail the need for more substantial SSDH content and tools, especially for the interprofessional teams. Opportunities involve centralized training, aligning educational/practice outcomes, and enhancing SSDH-related learning and resources. Threats encompass constraints on provider time, motivation, and community resource awareness.

IMPLICATIONS

Recognizing and tackling SSDH within clinical practice can yield profound and beneficial effects on patient outcomes, health care delivery, and the holistic wellness of individuals and communities. Health care providers can better support patients by engaging in accessible and continuous staff education about SSDH and on-going professional development on how to implement SSDH into practice. Health care providers can also better support patients facing social challenges by inquiring about their social history, offering guidance, connecting them with local support services, facilitating access to these services, and serving as a reliable source of information. One practical approach to achieve these goals is to integrate screening protocols into clinical practice. SSDH screening entails methodically evaluating the social and environmental factors that can influence patients' health outcomes. This process should be followed by providing accessible community resources to address the identified determinants. A first step in this process is culturally sensitive questioning about potential social challenges. Implementing SSDH screening has the potential to enhance patient care and mitigate health inequities.

Nurses encounter patients throughout the care continuum and consider each patient's needs to ensure successful health outcomes. Regular SSDH screening assists health care providers to assess and address unmet social needs directly impacting patient health. Factors like economic status, housing stability, and access to healthy food are systematically evaluated, revealing underlying determinants affecting health. Armed with this information, health care professionals can customize interventions, addressing root causes, not just symptoms, resulting in more effective and comprehensive care. SSDH screening promotes patient-centered care by recognizing unique contexts, preferences, and challenges that shape each individual's health journey. This approach fosters tailored care plans, collaboration, and empowerment, enhancing patient engagement and well-being while improving treatment adherence and health outcomes.

SSDH screening aligns with efforts to reduce health inequities by addressing social and economic determinants of health. Expanding access to quality behavioral health services is essential for providing whole-person care and improving SSDH outcomes. Health equity, encompassing behavioral health and SSDH factors, are interconnected. By recognizing and addressing these underlying determinants, health care providers actively work toward dismantling barriers that disproportionately affect underrepresented and underserved populations. SSDH screening reveals inequities among demographic groups, enabling targeted interventions to close health outcome gaps. This promotes equitable resource distribution and reduces historical inequities. Embracing SSDH screening reflects a commitment to social justice, ensuring equal access to health opportunities. It identifies inequities and lays the foundation for targeted interventions, fostering a more equitable health care landscape.

CONCLUSION AND CALL TO ACTION

In the pursuit of holistic and patient-centered care, nurses find themselves at a critical juncture. Serving as frontline health care providers, nurses possess a unique opportunity to profoundly influence the lives of patients beyond their medical treatment. By recognizing the significance of SSDH, nurses can proactively take steps to address these factors within their clinical practice.

Nurses can make a profound impact on the lives of those they care for through their unwavering commitment, empathy, and dedication. When nurses actively address SSDH, they can dismantle barriers, mitigate health inequities, and contribute to a more equitable health care system, ultimately shaping a healthier future for individuals and communities. Equipped with a comprehensive and up-to-date directory of community resources, nurses can acquire valuable insights into problem-specific referral options available in their local area. Nurses, as both health care providers and advocates for positive change, should wholeheartedly embrace the task of assessing and addressing SSDH within their clinical practice.

Nurses can further impact the lives of those they serve by disseminating evidence-based interventions, policies, and practices that form the foundation of health care quality and shape outcomes in both academic and clinical settings. It's crucial to have a deep understanding of and advocate for policies that promote equitable health care. By disseminating information about how educational and clinical programs address and support policies related to equitable health care, nurses can play a role in shaping policy decisions. This dissemination can also enhance policymakers' awareness, knowledge, and motivation to translate research findings into actionable policies, creating an environment conducive to adopting equity-focused initiatives. Moreover, addressing the issue of low knowledge and limited beliefs about health inequities among providers, emerging health care professionals, and policymakers is essential. By disseminating practice interventions across various health care settings, we can promote a better understanding of how to implement and promote best practices that facilitate the adoption of evidence-based information and ultimately advance equitable health care solutions.

Challenging Thoughts to Consider

1. Detail the steps to strategize how a nurse practitioner would incorporate the concept of person-centered care into a nursing practice model of health care delivery that reflects caring, quality, safety, efficiency, and equity.

2. Explore the integration of SSDH into health care, educational, and clinical settings with a broader focus on the impact of working with systems and agencies. How and when should this integration occur to ensure health care providers will accept and utilize the knowledge and tools to deliver comprehensive care?

3. Discuss the variability of creating sustainable infrastructure and workflow needs for social interactions to advocate for social change to address health inequities.

References

Alderwick, H., & Gottlieb, L. M. (2019). Meanings and misunderstandings: a social determinants of health lexicon for health care systems. *The Milbank Quarterly, 97*(2), 407–419. https://doi.org/10.1111/1468-0009.12390

Alegría, M., NeMoyer, A., Falgàs Bagué, I., Wang, Y., & Alvarez, K. (2018). Social determinants of mental health: where we are and where we need to go. *Current Psychiatry Reports, 20*(11), 95. https://doi.org/10.1007/s11920-018-0969-9

Andermann, A. (2018). Screening for social determinants of health in clinical care: moving from the margins to mainstream. *Public Health Reviews, 39*, 19. https://doi.org/10.1186/s40985-018-0094-7

Artiga, S., & Hinton, E. (2018). *Beyond health care: the role of social determinants in promoting health and health equity*. http://www.

ccapcomcare.org/Newsletters/2018-05%20 INSIGHT%20KFF%20Brief.pdf

Bechtel, N., Jones, A., Kue, J., & Ford, J. L. (2022). Evaluation of the core 5 social determinants of health screening tool. *Public Health Nursing*, *39*, 438–445. https://doi.org/10.1111/phn.12983

Billioux, A., Verlander, K., Anthony, S., & Alley, D. (2017). *Standardized screening for health-related social needs in clinical settings: the accountable health communities screening tool*. NAM Perspectives. https://doi.org/10.31478/201705b

Boss, R., & Gulley, J. (2022). *Behavioral health equity for all communities: policy solutions to advance equity across the crisis continuum*. National Governors Association Center for Best Practices and Technical Assistance Collaborative.

Bradywood, A., Leming-Lee, T., Watters, R., & Blackmore, C. (2021). Implementing screening for social determinants of health using the Core 5 tool. *BMJ Open Quality*, *10*, e001362. https://doi.org/10.1136/bmjoq-2021-001362

Braveman, P., Egerter, S., & Williams, D. R. (2011). The social determinants of health: Coming of age. *Annual Review of Public Health*, *32*, 381–398. https://doi.org/10.1146/annurev-publhealth-031210-101218

Braveman, P., & Gottlieb, L. (2014). The social determinants of health; It's time to consider the causes of the causes. *Public Health Records*, *129*(Suppl 2), 19–31. https://doi.org/10.1177/00333549141291S206

Center for Practice Innovations. (2024). https://www.practiceinnovations.org/

Chepaitis, A., Kordomenos, C., Bernacet, A. (2021, April 16). Social determinants of health: Language nuance matters. RTI International. https://www.rti.org/insights/key-concepts-in-social-determinants-of-health

Counts, N. (2023, May). *Understanding the U.S. Behavioral Health Workforce Shortage (explainer)*. Commonwealth Fund. https://doi.org/10.26099/5km6-8193

County Health Rankings & Roadmaps. (2022). University of Wisconsin Population Health Institute. https://www.countyhealthrankings.org

Davis, S. (2022). The evolving role of social determinants of health too advance health equity. In Seibert, Malone, & DeLeon (Eds). *Shaping nursing healthcare policy: A View from the Inside*. (pp. 1–102). Academic Press.

de Mooij, L. D., Kikkert, M., Theunissen, J., Beekman, A. T. F., de Haan, L., Duurkoop, P. W. R. A., Van, H. L., & Dekker, J. J. M. (2019). Dying too soon: excess mortality in severe mental illness. *Frontiers in Psychiatry*, *10*, 855. https://doi.org/10.3389/fpsyt.2019.00855

Deferio, J. J., Breitinger, S., Khullar, D., Sheth, A., & Pathak, J. (2019). Social determinants of health in mental health care and research: a case for greater inclusion. *Journal of the American Medical Informatics Association (JAMIA)*, *26*(8–9), 895–899. https://doi.org/10.1093/jamia/ocz049

Gattu, R. K., Paik, G., Wang, Y., Ray, P., Lichenstein, R., & Black, M. M. (2019). The hunger vital sign identifies household food insecurity among children in emergency departments and primary care. *Children*, *6*(10), 107. https://doi.org/10.3390/children6100107

Green, K., & Zook, M. (2019, October 29). When talking about social determinants of health, precision matters. *Health Affairs*. https://www.healthaffairs.org/do/10.1377/forefront.20191025.776011/

Heath, S. (2020, February 26). *Action needed for social determinants of Health, Health Equity*. Patient Engagement HIT. https://patientengagementhit.com/news/action-needed-for-social-determinants-of-health-health-equity

Kaiser Permanente. (2019). *Kaiser Permanente research: Social needs in America*. Kaiser Permanente Center for Health Research. https://about.kaiserpermanente.org/content/dam/internet/kp/comms/import/uploads/2019/06/KP-Social-Needs-Survey-Key-Findings.pdf

Khan, M., Ilcisin, M., & Saxton, K. (2017). Multifactorial discrimination as a fundamental cause of mental health inequities. *International Journal for Equity in Health*. https://doi.org/10.1186/s12939-017-0532-z

McKnight-Eily, L. R., Okoro, C. A., Strine, T. W., Verlenden, J., Hollis, N. D., Njai, R.,

Mitchell, E. W., Board, A., Puddy, R., & Thomas, C. (2021). Racial and ethnic disparities in the prevalence of stress and worry, mental health conditions, and increased substance use among adults during the COVID-19 pandemic—United States, April and May 2020. *MMWR. Morbidity and Mortality Weekly Report, 70*(5), 162–166. https://doi.org/10.15585/mmwr.mm7005a3

Muirhead, L., Brasher, S., Broadnax, D., & Chandler, R. (2022). A framework for evaluating SDH curriculum integration. *Journal of Professional Nursing, 39*, 1–9. https://doi.org/10.1016/j.profnurs.2021.12.004

National Academies of Science, Engineering, and Medicine. (NASEM). (2017). Communities in action: Pathways to health equity. Exploring the root causes of heath inequity. https://nap.nationalacademies.org/resource/24624/RootCausesofHealthInequity/

National Academies of Sciences, Engineering, and Medicine (NASEM). (2021). "3. The nursing workforce." *The Future of Nursing 2020–2030: Charting a Path to Achieve Health Equity*. Washington, DC: The National Academies Press. https://doi.org/10.17226/25982.

National League for Nursing (NLN). (2019). *A vision for integration of the social determinants of health into nursing education curricula: A living document from the national league for nursing, NLN Vision Series*. http://www.nln.org/docs/default-source/default-documentlibrary/social-determinants-of-health.pdf?sfvrsn=2

New York State Office of Mental Health. (n.d.) https://omh.ny.gov/

NIDA. (2022, September 27). *Part 1: The connection between substance use disorders and mental illness.* https://nida.nih.gov/publications/research-reports/common-comorbidities-substance-use-disorders/part-1-connection-between-substance-use-disorders-mental-illness

Page-Reeves, J., Kaufman, W., Bleecker, M., Norris, J., McCalmont, K., Ianakieva, V., Ianakieva, D., & Kaufman, A. (2016). Addressing social determinants of health in a clinic setting: the WellRX pilot in Albuquerque, New Mexico. *Journal of American Board of Family Medicine, 29*(3), 414–418. https://doi.org/10.3122/jabfm.2016.03.150272

Pevalin, D. J., Reeves, A., Baker, E., & Bentley, R. (2017). The impact of persistent poor housing conditions on mental health: a longitudinal population-based study. *Preventive Medicine, 105*, 304–310. https://doi.org/10.1016/j.ypmed.2017.09.020

Ray, R., Lantz, P. M., & Williams, D. (2023). Upstream policy changes to improve population health and health equity: A priority agenda. *The Milbank Quarterly, 101*(S1), p. 20–35.

Shim, R. S., & Compton, M. T. (2018). Addressing the social determinants of mental health: If not now, when? If not us, who? *Psychiatric Services (Washington, D.C.), 69*(8), 844–846. https://doi.org/10.1176/appi.ps.201800060

Substance Abuse and Mental Health Services Administration (SAMHSA). (2021). *Key substance use and mental health indicators in the United States: Results from the 2020 national survey on drug use and health* (HHS Publication No. PEP21-07-01-003, NSDUH Series H-56). Center for Behavioral Health Statistics and Quality, Substance Abuse and Mental Health Services Administration. https://www.samhsa.gov/data/

The health leads screening toolkit. (2018). https://healthleadsusa.org/communications-center/resources/the-health-leads-screening-toolkit/

The Root Cause Coalition. (2020). *State of Health Equity Report*. https://7862fdfe-0556-4f23-ac6f-74a72ae13c27.usrfiles.com/ugd/15441f_6af22d11f5f846eab5841eef847d1c29.pdf

Thornton, M., & Persaud, S. (2018). Preparing today's nurses: social determinants of health and nursing education. *OJIN: The Online Journal of Issues in Nursing, 23*(3). https://doi.org/10.3912/OJIN.Vol23No03Man05

U.S. Census Bureau. (2023). *U.S. Census Bureau QuickFacts: New York*. https://www.census.gov/quickfacts/fact/table/NY/PST045222

Wark, K., Woodbury, R. B., LaBrie, S., Trainor, J., Freeman, M., & Avey, J. P. (2022). Engaging stakeholders in social determinants of health quality improvement efforts. *The Permanente Journal*, *26*, 28–38.

Weir, R. C., Proser, M., Jester, M., Li, V., Hood-Ronick, C. M., & Gurewich, D. (2020). Collecting social determinants of health data in the clinical setting: findings from National PRAPARE Implementation. *Journal of Health Care for the Poor and Underserved*, *31*(2), 1018–1035. https://doi.org/10.1353/hpu.2020.0075

Wyse, R., Hwang, W. T., Ahmed, A. A., Richards, E., & Deville, C., Jr. (2020). Diversity by race, ethnicity, and sex within the U.S. psychiatry physician workforce. *Academic Psychiatry the Journal of the American Association of Directors of Psychiatric Residency Training and the Association for Academic Psychiatry*, *44*(5), 523–530. https://doi.org/10.1007/s40596-020-01276-z

3

Partnerships: Community Engagement in Social Determinants of Health

Phyllis D. Morgan, PhD, FNP-BC, CNE, FAANP
Megan L. Jester, PhD, RN, AHN-BC
Deborah Finn-Romero, DNP, RN, PHN, PACT

INTRODUCTION

This chapter highlights examples of collaborative partnerships aimed at collectively improving community health outcomes. According to the *Future of Nursing* (NASEM, 2021) report, multisector partnerships play a crucial role in advancing health equity. These partnerships extend beyond traditional health care organizations and encompass a wide range of stakeholders, including schools, housing agencies, faith-based institutions, essential businesses, government agencies, nonprofit organizations, and more. The scope of these partnerships may involve various activities, such as consulting with community experts, educational training, service-learning opportunities, gathering input from stakeholders, providing wrap-around services, and contributing to policy development. Effective facilitation and coordination of these partnerships demand relationship-building, collaboration, trust-building, and a long-term shared commitment among all involved parties. Well-organized and engaged partnerships, with a strong focus on meeting the specific needs of a community, can effectively address social and structural determinants of health (SSDH) and contribute to improving health equity.

Values and Alignment

The understanding of SSDH emphasizes the imperative to collaborate in enhancing community health outcomes. The interconnected nature of the problems affecting our society means that they rarely have an isolated solution. Just as human well-being thrives on connections with others, organizations must also foster relationships to thrive.

The formation of partnerships, particularly those geared toward the health and well-being of all individuals, is fundamental for the future of our society and the world. Like unique human cultures, each organizational culture must identify common ground, shared goals, and mutual benefits in the creation of partnerships. Establishing trust, clarifying identifying goals and outcomes, and defining roles are the initial steps in collaborative work.

The Leadership Academy has highlighted the benefits of both traditional and nontraditional partnerships as effective means of enhancing health outcomes. The underlying philosophy is based on addressing complex issues collectively for the well-being of all society members through individual and multisector partnerships. This chapter embodies our commitment to working cooperatively with all individuals and organizations to address current and future sources of harm, such as racism, discrimination, economic disparity, religious intolerance, and gender bias.

Chapter Objectives

Upon completion of this chapter, the learner will be able to:

1. Foster a deeper understanding of collaborative partnerships that transcend traditional health care institutions, emphasizing their critical role in enhancing community health outcomes and addressing SSDH.

2. Identify the skills and knowledge necessary for effective facilitation and coordination of multisector partnerships by focusing on relationship-building, collaboration strategies, trust-building, and the establishment of long-term commitments among diverse stakeholders.

3. Explore practical approaches and strategies employed by successful partnerships in meeting community-specific needs and advancing health equity, drawing insights from case studies and real-world examples.

BACKGROUND

Identifying common goals and value-based outcomes forms the foundation for partnership development (Blank, 2015). According to Blank (2015), it is advisable to begin by identifying the data and interests that hold significance for each partner. Moreover, considerations, such as examining past events, successful strategies, and understanding barriers and challenges can provide valuable insights for future endeavors (Blank, 2015). Community issues and problems are complex, inextricably linked, and systemic, requiring broad viewpoints and interprofessional interventions through collaborative partnerships.

Partnerships can originate and develop from various avenues and across different sectors of society. Governmental agencies, for-profit and nonprofit businesses, clinical organizations, faith-based institutions, community organizations, educational institutions, and others represent viable options for successful partnerships. Collaborative ventures between organizations can yield benefits, such as cost-sharing and increased impact, ultimately serving the needs of the community more effectively (Emery et al., 2023). Partnerships focused on improving community outcomes manifest in several ways. Interprofessional partnerships represent involvement from several professional disciplines, working together to address complex issues. Professionals may come from similar sectors, such as health care or expand across sectors.

Multisector partnerships represent collaborations that expand beyond a single section of society. These partnerships may involve governments, nonprofit organizations, for-profit businesses, academic institutions, community stakeholders, and others, all focused and committed to addressing a complex issue. Partners may be engaged in direct work with the community or working in the background on financial needs, policy formation, and other strategic planning aspects. Multisector community partnerships have the capacity to solve systemic issues because they gather resources from multiple entities. Both interprofessional and multisector community partnerships play a pivotal role in advancing the health and well-being of our populations, as they enable more substantial achievements compared to individual organizational efforts (Willis et al., 2017).

Academic partnerships are collaborations that occur between educational institutions. Academic institutions often lead the way for change within society through new discovery, dissemination, and collaborative partnerships with all sectors of society. Partnerships include any level of education and varying areas of specialty and study. Research-based universities and colleges' primary mission is focused on innovation, discovery, and the translation of knowledge. Teaching-focused colleges and universities are mainly engaged in the sharing of knowledge for practice. Both types of institutions function with research and dissemination of knowledge but will have one or the other as the focus. Student experiences in a variety of educational settings allow for a broader viewpoint, opportunities for expanded knowledge within a chosen field, and opportunities to practice newly acquired skills. This Leadership Academy is an example of an academic-association partnership, bringing educators together from research, policy, and teaching-focused institutions for the purpose of expanding and sharing knowledge on SSDH, as well as SSDH's implications and strategies to improve communities' and populations' health and well-being.

Key components for building successful partnerships include the following: focusing on common goals, clearly defining roles and expectations, obtaining input from stakeholders, ensuring mutual benefits, and sharing responsibility for desired outcomes. Trust is fundamental to partnership development, and it involves staff interaction, learning, mutual support, leadership support in terms of resources, and a shared understanding (Naleppa & Waldbillig, 2018; Potts-Datema et al., 2005). The existing literature contains numerous studies highlighting multisector partnerships, which are recognized as a public health and SSDH strategy for achieving the common goal of community well-being (Emery et al., 2023).

Stakeholder participation is a fundamental component of any successful partnership. Stakeholders encompass individuals or groups with interests or those who will be affected by the proposed work. This includes leaders of all involved organizations responsible for resource allocation and individuals who stand to benefit from the work, including community members. Organizing publicized and inclusive stakeholder meetings is essential for introducing the project or intervention and listening to the thoughts, ideas, and considerations of all involved, regardless of their roles in the project. During these initial stages, designers must remain flexible to adapt plans based on the expressed needs and concerns of the stakeholders.

It is advisable to initiate discussions with individuals who are the primary focus of any intervention right from the initial planning stages. Similar to community-based participatory research, individuals should have a voice in what is being planned for them or on their behalf. In fact, their insights regarding their needs may differ significantly from the perspectives of outsiders looking into their community. These individuals or populations should be considered the foremost stakeholders in any project, and their input should be carefully considered before finalizing the intervention. As emphasized in all multisector partnerships, the establishment of trust is crucial for the success of any endeavor.

MULTISECTOR INSTITUTIONAL PARTNERSHIPS: POTENTIAL AGENCIES
Government Agencies

On a global level, the World Health Organization (WHO, 2023) is actively engaged in cross-border collaborations, addressing public health needs in both the public and private sectors. Blanchet et al. (2014) highlight a growing need for developing nations to receive support, both in core health assistance and secondary financial support, through collaborations with other nations. The significance of intersectoral collaborations is also recognized on a national level. As stated in *The Role of Public-Private Partnerships in Strengthening Health Systems*, partnerships across sectors are vital because health is a collective responsibility, and the complexity of health issues demands collective action (IHME, 2010). Although the United States (U.S.) government has a history of public-private sector partnerships, the focus on health is gaining prominence. The U.S. Interagency Council on Homelessness (USICH), comprising 19 U.S. government agencies, was established in 1987 to address homelessness and houselessness. Over the decades, it has evolved to prioritize transitioning unhoused individuals into permanent housing and addressing homelessness-related traumas (United States Interagency Council on Homelessness, n.d.). The agency offers toolkits and partnership models for addressing the health needs of those without housing, such as the Medicaid Innovation Accelerator Program State Medicaid-Housing Agency Partnerships Toolkit (United States Interagency Council on Homelessness, 2019). Local governments aligned with USICH initiatives are encouraged to collaborate with community organizations to develop and implement programs.

Recognizing the increasing health and economic needs, several other U.S. government agencies are expanding their multisector partnership initiatives to address the complex health needs of society. Collaboration between organizations is now a mandatory criterion for many federal grant applications. For instance, the U.S. Department of Labor's grant program for nursing expansion stipulates that applicants must partner at a minimum with four organizations, including non-profit health care agencies, educational institutions, labor unions, and workforce development leadership groups (U.S. Department of Labor, 2022). Federal grant initiatives are placing significant emphasis on tackling issues related to SSDH that impact vulnerable populations. *Healthy People 2030*, an initiative of the U.S. Department of Health and Human Services, highlights that many key health indicators and core measurements for the nation's health are centered around SSDH (Medicaid Innovation Accelerator Program, 2019).

In the U.S., governments frequently collaborate with community partners to support various directives and mandated initiatives. These government partnerships take on various forms. Federal partnerships, for instance, often offer grant funding opportunities, covering academic research, community programs, or private contracts. Eligibility for these grants can extend to state, county, and city governments, as well as private for-profit and nonprofit organizations, depending on the grant's terms and criteria. Similar opportunities for grants may also originate from state, county, and city governments, which may extend these grants to private organizations. Additionally, project-based collaborations with governmental bodies outside the scope of grants are possible. These collaborations are often driven by city, county, or state initiatives, leading organizations to apply for contracts that support mandated actions. Another notable form of governmental collaboration occurs with educational institutions. These partnerships encompass various activities, such as internships, specialized graduate projects, and mentorship programs, often as part of degree requirements. Each collaborating organization typically formalizes these arrangements with a Memorandum of Understanding (MOU), which serves as a contractual agreement outlining the partnership's requirements and terms.

Government partnerships can be either ongoing or limited term, often focusing on projects driven by administrative mandates. One notable example is the partnership between the U.S. Department of Housing and Urban Development (HUD) and organizations at the county level through the Continuum of Care (CoC) program. This multisector initiative is active in every county nationwide and aims to end homelessness, reduce homelessness-related trauma, and promote self-sufficiency among those experiencing homelessness (Housing and Urban Development, 2023). Partnering agencies are typically nonprofit organizations operating in accordance with grant funding regulations aligned with the CoC's mission.

Nonprofit Agencies

Nonprofit agencies that focus on enhancing society's well-being often make excellent partners for supporting SSDH initiatives. Organizations that typically qualify for nonprofit status include those with charitable, educational, faith-based, or community well-being objectives. However, not all entities under these designations choose to operate as nonprofits; some maintain for-profit status with government authorities. To achieve nonprofit status, an organization must apply to the Internal Revenue Service, which assesses whether it meets the necessary criteria. Nonprofit agencies can receive funds and donations from various sources, including for-profit entities, government agencies, and private donors. It is crucial that all funds received by the organization are used to further its stated mission to maintain nonprofit status.

Nonprofit Community Agencies

Nonprofit community agencies often make willing and capable partners for supporting SSDH initiatives at the local level. These socially focused organizations inherently recognize gaps in the capacity of governments and larger entities to directly engage with individuals in need. They rely on donations and grant awards that align with their organizational missions, typically resulting in narrow operating budgets staffed by dedicated professionals. The SSDH community initiatives that target neighborhoods and built environments, economic resources, educational programs, health care access, and social contexts are all suitable for partnerships with these smaller, multisector organizations.

BOX 3.1

Exemplar 1: Multisector Partnership, Permanent Housing for Persons Experiencing Homelessness

Persons who experience homelessness (PEH) for one year or more are considered the most vulnerable in society. Lack of resources across the SSDH domains for extended lengths of time leave many such individuals feeling rejected by society, with little hope of regaining stability. Through multisector partnerships, the development of wrap-around programs provides an opportunity to create new stability for PEH. Housing First initiatives are recommended by the United States Interagency Council on Homelessness (United States Interagency Council on Homelessness, 2015), as the first step in a multifactored approach to resolve the homeless crisis.

Sacramento County, in cooperation with cross-sector agencies and businesses, developed a permanent, supportive housing program for PEH referred to as Flexible, Supportive Rehousing Program (FSRP), now referred to as the Flexible Housing Pool (FHP) (Sacramento County, 2019 & 2023). The development of the program was modeled after Los Angeles County's Housing First model, Housing for Health (Rand, 2017).

The FHP program requires intensive support for the clients through Intensive Case Management Services (ICMS). These case managers are employed within nonprofit organizations contracting with the county to serve as the PEH's navigator toward reestablishing stability and health.

A training program was developed in cooperation with a doctoral student to prepare case managers for all aspects of the role. On the basis of significant evaluation of Housing First research, and community stakeholder input and participation from 14 independent agencies, the comprehensive program was delivered over several weeks. Topics covered the scope and perspective of the unhoused crisis nationally and locally, crisis intervention, motivational interviewing, cultural humility, gender and sexuality, disparity and stigma, sex offenders, substance use and dependency, mental and physical health, women's needs, dependent adults, and other topics. Government agencies from both Sacramento County and City, nonprofit social service organizations, private counselors, state policy legislative advocacy groups, private safety organizations, universities, nonprofit legal services, nurses, health care agencies, and others contributed to the development and delivery of content to the Intensive Case Management Services (ICMS) team (Finn-Romero, 2022).

Nongovernmental Organizations

Nongovernmental organizations (NGOs) are typically large entities with significant societal impacts at local, national, and international levels. They often operate as nonprofit organizations, managing annual budgets that can reach into the billions of dollars. Well-known examples of NGOs include The Red Cross, Amnesty International, Unicef, and Doctors Without Borders (United Nations Department of Economic and Social Affairs: Disability, n.d.). These organizations frequently collaborate with local and national government agencies to provide aid during humanitarian crises or when large-scale interventions are required. See Box 3.1.

ACADEMIC PARTNERSHIPS

K–12 Schools and Universities in the Community

Collaboration between educational institutions involves both academic entities working together to achieve a broader mission of addressing SSDH and collaboratively creating mutual learning opportunities. This partnership raises questions about resource sharing, mutual benefits, and what unique contributions each institution can offer to effectively serve the communities in need. Academic institutions have a responsibility to address SSDH through research, practice, education, and foster interprofessional collaboration, interprofessional education, and interprofessional practice.

Addressing SSDH necessitates a concerted effort from both health care institutions and school communities. Emphasizing equity through the integration of health care and education access within SSDH is crucial for students' success (Blank, 2015). Health-related issues among children and adolescents can lead to chronic absenteeism, behavioral challenges, and academic setbacks (Blank, 2015). Mental health concerns stand out as a leading cause of adverse outcomes in young individuals in the U.S. ("Protecting youth mental health," 2021). Schools are increasingly becoming primary settings to identify and address students' mental health needs (Christian & Brown, 2018). Moreover, the COVID-19 pandemic underscored the pivotal role of schools in the social and emotional development of young people, revealing the consequences when this support is lacking. The importance of addressing SSDH and health equity through school-based partnerships is highlighted in the *Future of Nursing 2020–2030* report by NASEM (2021), the National Institute of Nursing Research's (NINR) 2022–2026 strategic plan and is a priority for several national organizations, including recognizing the critical role of school nurses at the intersection of health care, education, and community (Best & McCabe, 2023; NASEM, 2021; NINR, 2022; Tanner & Stanislo, 2022).

Community engagement is a fundamental aspect of developing partnerships with academic and educational institutions, yielding mutual benefits (McMullen et al., 2020). These advantages encompass increased access to resources, a sense of communal purpose and empowerment, and valuable service-learning opportunities (McMullen et al., 2020). Academic and educational institutions serve as critical conduits for preparing students to address SSDH. According to Hassan and Bui (2022), educational interventions provide essential strategies for equipping learners with the tools needed to effect change in clinical practice. Hassan and Bui (2022) have outlined a framework for integrating structurally competent clinical reasoning into case-based presentations. It is imperative to incorporate structural competency curricula into undergraduate and graduate education programs. This framework involves four key steps: 1) developing a prioritized clinical program, 2) identifying root causes of clinical problems in terms of structural determinants of health, 3) constructing a prioritized structural list, and 4) brainstorming to formulate solutions to address structural issues (Hassan & Bui, 2022). Thus, students should be adequately prepared in the domain of structural competency.

Case studies are frequently employed to impart critical thinking skills to students, teaching them how to address SSDH. Page's (2010) model is a well-known approach for crafting unfolding case studies. However, this raises the question of whether there should be a specialized model designed explicitly for case studies aimed at fostering critical thinking regarding SSDH. Hekel et al. (2023) discovered that unfolding case studies can serve as potent tools for integrating SSDH into education and patient care. These case studies effectively teach clinical judgment and prepare students for the Next Generation NCLEX.

Success in addressing SSDH must extend beyond the conventional school day and takes commitment and shared goals. There are barriers to consider, such as budget constraints, the time required for nurturing relationships, and the risk of excluding parental or caregiver involvement, all of which can influence student success (Sauder et al., 2017). Blank (2015) put forth four key factors that positively impact school-based health partnerships. First, shared ownership involves the equal allocation of resources and shared responsibility for outcomes, fostering relationship growth (Blank, 2015). Second, innovation spreading, including how students access services, promotes equity in health care and education access (Blank, 2015). Third, there's a need for deep changes in the mindset of all parties involved, addressing perceptions, biases, stereotypes, and expectations (Blank, 2015). Finally, sustainable school-based partnerships require the establishment of an infrastructure encompassing emotional, financial, physical, and verbal support. This support should be coupled with a strategic, time-bound measurement of progress and a clear vision and purpose (Blank, 2015). By applying these factors, school-based partnerships can lead to improved student health and educational outcomes, ultimately contributing to progress toward health equity for all students. See Box 3.2.

BOX 3.2

Exemplar 2: Pre-Kindergarten Through 12th Grade School Partnerships

Understanding how SSDH impacts a child's emotional and physical safety at the beginning of their school day is essential. Consequently, a school-based partnership was established in the Midwestern U.S., involving three university programs: nursing, educational psychology, and interior design, in collaboration with a large urban elementary school that faces social and structural inequities. The primary aim of this partnership was to identify shared research priorities and develop programs to evaluate the school's physical environment. The focus was on understanding the school's current infrastructure and its role during students' morning transition, from their arrival at the school to their classroom, where they participate in a class-wide morning meeting designed to regulate social and emotional behaviors and autonomic function.

Relationship building took place over a span of 1.5 years to establish trust with school administrators, the school nurse, and other staff members. This involved providing interprofessional health education to students and families at health fairs and parent-teacher conferences, as well as participating in various strategic planning meetings. To establish baseline building attributes, three-dimensional scanning will be conducted for spatial and physical measurements, while photovoice will be used to capture student perspectives. Structured and unstructured drawings will be employed to elicit students' ideal perceptions of a supportive physical environment for their psychosocial awareness. Interviews with school staff will provide insights into their perceptions of student behavior and their assessment of physical and emotional safety. Additionally, autonomic function will be measured upon students' arrival in their classroom, with an early focus on understanding the impact of SSDH on blood pressure and heart rate. This initiative offers a valuable, innovative opportunity to develop school-based partnerships that prioritize the emotional and physical safety of children through the assessment and design of the built environment. This unique collaboration between nursing, educational psychology, and interior design will contribute significantly to comprehending the influence of SSDH on the built environment, promoting equity in health care and educational access for Pre-K through 12th-grade students, and fostering equitable policy development and building design.

Partnerships With Historically Black Colleges and Universities

Partnerships between Historically Black Colleges and Universities (HBCUs) and Predominantly White Institutions (PWIs) become feasible when there is a clear understanding of resource capacity, sustainability, and scholarly objectives (Warren et al., 2019). There can be ambivalence on both sides, with HBCUs and PWIs questioning who stands to benefit from such a partnership and how these institutions, representing different demographic majorities and minorities, will derive value from it. These partnerships have emerged in response to the pressing need for a racially and ethnically diverse health care workforce (Jae et al., 2021). Innovative partnerships with HBCUs that surround interprofessional education and integrate SSDH can have a positive impact on diversity and equity in the health care profession (Holton et al., 2023). See Box 3.3.

BOX 3.3

Exemplar 3: Partnerships With Historically Black Colleges and Universities

Walden University, a prominent online institution, stands out with its mission to drive positive social change. This unique mission opens global opportunities for partnerships aimed at addressing SSDH. Notably, Walden University boasts a remarkable record of graduating a substantial number of doctoral degree recipients from diverse backgrounds, making it a global leader in this regard. Moreover, the university's largest academic program, nursing, plays a pivotal role in workforce diversity. On the other hand, Hampton University School of Nursing has a historic legacy as the first HBCU to offer a Doctor of Philosophy in Nursing. Both Walden University's College of Nursing and Hampton University share a common commitment to promoting diversity, equity, inclusion, and addressing SSDH.

Walden University College of Nursing and Hampton University School of Nursing initiated a collaborative partnership aimed at addressing SSDH & Social Change through faculty development and curriculum integration. A member of the National League for Nursing (NLN) and Walden University College of Nursing Social Determinants of Health & Social Change Leadership Academy spearheaded this project. Recognizing the need for faculty development in integrating SSDH into nursing curriculum, academic leaders from both institutions devised a three-fold approach: 1) a certificate program, 2) curriculum development, and 3) community application. This approach formed the foundation of this collaboration. The partnership's primary objectives encompass faculty development, scholarly pursuits, and the seamless integration of SSDH into the curriculum. To introduce this endeavor, a joint webinar was hosted during the Walden University National Faculty Meeting in the summer of 2023. The webinar served as a platform to showcase the collaborative efforts between Walden University College of Nursing and Hampton University School of Nursing, outlining their strategies for addressing SSDH through faculty development and an innovative curriculum. This partnership is a significant step toward promoting positive social change in the field of nursing education.

Community Faith-Based Organizations

Community and faith-based organizations are crucial in tackling SSDH and reducing health inequities (Manjunath et al., 2019). Successful partnerships between these organizations and health care initiatives exist, highlighting their potential impact. Faith-based

BOX 3.4

Exemplar 4: Community Education in Faith-Based Settings

Research demonstrates that cancer mortality rates are disproportionately high among African Americans compared to other ethnic groups. Identifying key stakeholders within the community is essential when establishing community or faith-based programs. Effective partnerships hinge on identifying and collaborating with individuals or organizations outside your own that share a vested interest in the initiative's success. Even if these external entities do not initially express interest, it is valuable to extend invitations for discussions on potential partnerships, as such collaborations can yield mutual benefits for both organizations.

Triple Negative Breast Cancer (TNBC) disproportionately affects Black women compared to women from other ethnic/racial groups. The National Coalition of 100 Black Women Prince William County Chapter, Inc. (NCBW-PWCC) received funding by the Potomac Health Foundation to implement a community/faith-based breast health educational focus on TNBC for Black women (Howard et al., 2016). The program's design was rooted in existing literature, which highlighted the effectiveness of faith-based educational initiatives in enhancing cancer awareness and encouraging screening behaviors. In this endeavor, community engagement was paramount. The goal was to create a community/faith-based initiative that would educate Black women about TNBC and promote regular mammography screenings among this demographic.

A multi-interprofessional approach was employed to execute a project focused on TNBC. The project team established a community advisory board, comprising nurses, advanced practice nurses, physicians, ministers, local hospital representatives, breast cancer survivors, political leaders, and community advocates for African American health issues. This advisory board convened monthly to review project advancements and verify that it aligned with the community's needs.

The project was meticulously designed to ensure cultural appropriateness for the target participants. Ministers offered prayers before and after culturally tailored community/faith-based educational programs on TNBC. The project featured African American health care providers, culturally relevant educational materials, specially crafted videos, and the inclusion of African American breast cancer survivors to facilitate its implementation. The community/faith-based educational program substantially enhanced the knowledge of Black women about TNBC and promoted increased mammography screening behaviors (Howard et al., 2016). Participants provided enthusiastic feedback and evaluations for the TNBC community/faith-based project. Consequently, the organization secured funding for additional initiatives aimed at enhancing awareness and screening behaviors for various cancers, including prostate cancer for Black men and a colorectal cancer program for both Black men and women. The organization successfully achieved its objectives to boost screening rates for breast, colorectal, and prostate cancer.

institutions can serve as valuable allies in supporting underserved communities. Often acting as community hubs, they foster a sense of belonging among culturally similar populations, addressing the social and community aspects of SSDH. These organizations can effectively reach specific demographic groups, making them valuable partners for targeted SSDH interventions. See Box 3.4.

Health Care Agency Partnerships

Health care agencies are increasingly realizing the importance of establishing community partnerships due to health care provider shortages and the complexities of

---

BOX 3.5

Exemplar 5: Health Care Agency Partnership

An organization received grant funding to educate the Black community about cancer and enhance cancer screenings. They used this opportunity to forge a valuable partnership with the local hospital to execute the grant's objectives. The hospital contributed essential resources to facilitate community/faith-based cancer education programs. These programs featured key presenters, including physicians, nurses, and nutritional experts, who were chosen to reflect the demographic makeup of the population being served. Extensive research has highlighted the positive impact of provider-patient relationships when health care providers share a similar ethnic or racial background with their patients (Snyder et al., 2023). In line with this, the hospital collaborated closely with our organization, providing the necessary resources and support to ensure the project's success. For instance, free mammograms were offered to Black women at the locations where educational programs were conducted. This collaboration helped to eliminate barriers to access and promote cancer screening in the Black community.

---

managing chronic and intricate health conditions (Green & Johnson, 2015; Hyochol et al., 2022). These collaborations offer numerous advantages, including reductions in emergency room visits and readmission rates. Collaborating with hospitals is particularly crucial in this regard. Hospitals have a vested interest in addressing SSDH for various reasons and actively engage in partnerships with community agencies to tackle these issues. Many hospitals have initiated community outreach programs aimed at assisting vulnerable and underserved populations and addressing SSDH. Moreover, health care agencies are establishing Diversity, Equity, and Inclusion centers to foster trust within the community, especially among Black and other historically excluded and underrepresented populations in underserved and underrepresented areas. These centers work toward enhancing health care access and addressing SSDH inequities. See Box 3.5.

Indigenous, First American, First Nations, Native American, Alaska Native Communities

Environmental factors and generational and historical trauma significantly influence the health outcomes of Indigenous Peoples, including American Indian, Alaska Native, and First American individuals and communities. For the purposes of this section, we will use the term "Indigenous" to encompass these groups. Overt harms, such as displacement, exploitation, and forced acculturation, have contributed to heightened health inequities within these communities. Moreover, the health inequities experienced by Indigenous populations are further exacerbated by the continued impact of historical harms combined with present-day inequities (e.g., food and health care access, chronic disease inequities) (Warne & Wescott, 2019) and limited understanding of these harms from non-Indigenous collaborators. It is crucial for non-Indigenous collaborators to recognize that they are engaging with sovereign nations when working with Indigenous communities, rather than merely interacting with different cultures (Jones et al., 2019, p. 488). Engagement appears as recognizing personal limitations, patience, active

> **BOX 3.6**
>
> ## Exemplar 6: Indigenous Community Partnerships
>
> A community-based approach was utilized to develop an after-school yoga program for school-age children at an urban Indigenous health care clinic. Multiple conversations occurred over the course of 1 year with key administrators in quality improvement and health promotion disease prevention, establishing a trusting, community-based relationship to design a culturally appropriate program. The conversations were based on listening to the needs of the clinic related to gaps in youth programming. The themes of each week's yoga session were developed collaboratively with the yoga participants, with emphasis on developing the sessions from an Indigenous worldview (e.g., kindness, giving thanks to nature). The approval process for the yoga program was multilayered within the clinic to ensure protection of the participants. Feedback from the participants was collected biweekly, to make necessary program revisions and for reports to clinic administration. This collaborative partnership increased access to physical activity for children and developed community-based partnership with high potential for sustainability.

listening, and demonstrating trustworthiness and follow-through (Jones et al., 2019). In developing partnerships, non-Indigenous collaborators must acknowledge the historical and ongoing harms faced by Indigenous populations and take proactive steps to avoid perpetuating these harms. This approach is essential for addressing the upstream determinants of SSDH and promoting health equity within Indigenous communities.

When collaborating with Indigenous communities, establishing strong relationships is not only a key consideration but also the foundational step to initiate any work (Gardner-Vandy & Scalice, 2020). For these collaborations to be effective, it is essential to prioritize building trust and rapport with Indigenous community members and leaders. Cultural adaptation is another crucial aspect of collaborating with Indigenous communities. Content or curriculum that is thoughtfully and respectfully tailored to the specific cultural context of an Indigenous community tends to have greater appeal and is better received (Sauder et al., 2017). This means considering the unique traditions, values, and worldviews of the community and incorporating them into the educational materials or programs being developed. Moreover, cultural adaptation demonstrates a commitment to cultural sensitivity and humility, which is vital when working with Indigenous populations. It shows respect for their cultural heritage and acknowledges the importance of preserving and promoting their traditions, while addressing pressing health and social issues. In summary, effective collaboration with Indigenous communities requires a foundation of trust and the development of culturally adapted materials and approaches to ensure that the work is relevant and respectful of the community's unique identity and needs, thereby promoting community-driven sustainability. See Box 3.6.

IMPLICATIONS

Partnerships are undeniably vital because they enable institutions and organizations to combine their resources, which can be particularly valuable in addressing the needs of individuals, families, and communities. Moreover, partnerships provide an opportunity to pool expertise, bringing together the knowledge and skills of various entities to tackle complex challenges effectively. When considering partnerships, it is crucial to conduct a thorough assessment, weighing the advantages and disadvantages. Ideally, the benefits of collaboration should outweigh any potential drawbacks. Partnerships come in various forms, driven by different motivations and objectives. What is paramount is ensuring that the partnership is aligned with the goal of addressing SSDH and that it mutually benefits all involved parties.

Recognizing that there are guidelines and established approaches for forming partnerships is key. Following these best practices can help ensure that the collaboration is well structured, productive, and sustainable. Importantly, many grant funding agencies now encourage and recommend collaborative approaches to address health issues. This reflects the recognition that tackling complex challenges like SSDH and health inequities often requires a multifaceted, interdisciplinary effort. In essence, addressing SSDH and eliminating health inequities cannot be achieved in isolation. Developing collaborative partnerships is at the core of strengthening existing relationships and establishing new ones, all with the common purpose of improving the overall well-being of individuals and communities.

CONCLUSION AND CALL TO ACTION

The NLN and Walden University College of Nursing allocate resources toward community initiatives aimed at addressing SSDH and fostering positive social change. Participation in the NLN and Walden University College of Nursing Social Determinants of Health & Social Change Leadership Institute was an eye-opener for our cohort, emphasizing the vital role of partnerships in tackling SSDH.

This partnership between the NLN and Walden University College of Nursing played a pivotal role in establishing the Social Determinants of Health & Social Change Leadership Institute. Partnerships can take shape in various ways, either formally through engagements with government agencies, nonprofit organizations, health care institutions, or clinical agencies, or informally over casual conversations, coffee meetings, or meals. Effective partnerships hinge on communication and a shared commitment to working for the greater good in addressing SSDH. In this chapter, we perceive leaders as developers of partnerships, emphasizing the need for proactive engagement in forming partnerships. Multiple partnerships may be necessary to comprehensively address SSDH issues. A crucial call to action is to educate both faculty and students in the art of partnership development. Continue reading to explore how partnerships are formed and the key principles involved in establishing and sustaining them. The social and structural determinants of health significantly influence health care inequities, making collaborative partnerships, encompassing education, research, and practice, indispensable for addressing SSDH.

Challenging Thoughts to Consider

1. What is the value of collaborative partnerships in the transformation of community health outcomes?
2. What value can be given by utilization of SSDH for effective facilitation and coordination of selected types of partnerships?

3. What type of examples represent the demonstrated and positive impact on specific community needs and contribute to improving health equity?

4. What actions should the nurse practitioner engage in, for the development and implementation of multisector partnerships with long-term community commitments to improve individual and community health outcomes?

References

Best, N. C., & McCabe, E. M. (2023). Learning from the past and moving forward: Implementing school nursing research priorities. *The Journal of School Nursing, 39*(1), 3–5. https://doi.org/10.1177/10598405221143495

Blanchet, N., Thomas, M., Atun, R., Jamison, D., Knaul, F., & Hechet, R. (2014). *Global collective action in health: The WDR+20 landscape of core and supportive functions.* WIDER Working Paper 2014/011. UNU-WIDER. https://doi.org/10.35188/UNU-WIDER/2014/732-5

Blank, M. (2015). Building sustainable health and education partnerships: Stories from local communities. *Journal of School Health, 85*, 810–816. https://doi.org/10.1111/josh.12311

Christian, D. D., & Brown, C. L. (2018). Recommendations for the role and responsibilities of school-based mental health counselors. *Journal of School-Based Counseling Policy and Evaluation, 1*, 26–39. https://www.umass.edu/schoolcounseling/JSCPE_cissue.php

Emery, K. J., Durocher, B., Arena, L. C., Glasgow, L., Bayer, E. M., Plescia, M., Holtgrave, P. L., & Hacker, K. (2023). Health departments' role in addressing social determinants of health in collaboration the multisector community partnerships. *Journal of Public Health Management Practice. 29*(1), 51–55.

Finn-Romero, D. (2022). Community partnerships: training case managers working with individuals experiencing chronic homelessness. *Interdisciplinary Journal of Partnership Studies, 9*(1), Article 8. https://doi.org/10.24926/ijps.v9i1.4651

Gardner-Vandy, K., & Scalice, D. (2020). Relationships first and always: A guide to collaborations with Indigenous communities. *2020 Planetary Science and Astrobiology Decadal Survey 2020–2030.* https://nnigovernance.arizona.edu/sites/nnigovernance.arizona.edu/files/resources/31617915926903.pdf

Green, B. N., & Johnson, C. D. (2015). Interprofessional collaboration in research, education, and clinical practice: working together for a better future. *Journal of Chiropractic Education, 29*, 1–10. https://doi.org/10.7899/JCE-14-36

Hassan, I. F., & Bui, T. (2022). The structural analysis: Incorporating structurally competent clinical reasoning into case-based presentations. *Journal of General Internal Medicine, 37*(13), 3465–3468. https://doi.org/10.1007/s11606-022-07751-7

Hekel, B. E., Pullia, B. C., Edwards, A. P., & Alexander, J. (2023). Teaching social determinants of health through an unfolding case study. *Nurse Educator, 48*(3), 137–141. https://doi.org/10.1097/NNE.0000000000001333

Holton, C., Banerjee, S., Morgan, P., McCune, N. M., Cook, A., Thomas, J., & Vesey, A. (2023). Centering health equity through the social determinants of health, interprofessional education, and sustainable partnerships with historically black colleges and universities: envisioning upstream and downstream impacts. *Creative Nursing, 29*, 1–11. https://doi.org/10.1177/1078453231212477

Housing and Urban Development. (2023). *Continuum of care (CoC) program.* https://www.hudexchange.info/programs/coc/

Howard, A., Morgan, P. D., Golesorkhi, N., Zuurbier, R., Fogel, J., Lively, M. R., Simmons, E. D., Polk, T. A., Haynes, L., Richardson, E., & Withers, D. H. (2016). A community/faith-based breast health educational program focused on increasing knowledge about triple negative breast cancer among black women in Prince William County and surrounding areas. *JOCEPS: The Journal of Chi Eta Phi Sorority*, *59*, 6–10.

Hyochol, A., Butts, B., Cottrell, D. B., Kesey, J., McNeill, C. C., Mumba, M. N., O'Brien, T., Reifsnider, E., & Reilly, C. M. (2022). Partnerships to improve social determinants of health, health equity, and health outcomes: An SNRS white paper. *Research in Nursing & Health*, *45*, 8–10. https://doi.org/10.1002/nur.22198

IHME (Institute for Health Metrics and Evaluation). 2010. *2010 Global burden of diseases, injuries, and risk factors study*. University of Washington.

Jae, G., Iledare, E., Ander, D., Wallenstein, J., Anachebe, N., Elks, M., Franks, N., White, M., Shayne, P., Henn, M., & Heron, S. (2021). A model partnership: Mentoring underrepresented students in medicine. (URiM) in emergency medicine. *Western Journal of Emergency Medicine: Integrating Emergency Care with Population*, *22*(2), 213–217.

Jones, E. J., Haozous, E., Larsson, L. S., & Moss, M. P. (2019). Perspectives on conducting research in Indian country. *Nursing Research*, *68*(6), 488–493. https://doi.org/10.1097/NNR.0000000000000379

Manjunath, C., Ifelayo, O., Jones, C., Washington, M., Shanedling, S., Williams, J., Patten, C. A., & Cooper, L. (2019). Addressing cardiovascular health disparities in Minnesota: Establishment of a community steering committee by FAITH! (Fostering African-American improvement in total health). *International Journal of Environmental Research and Public Health*, *16*(21), 4144. https://doi.org/10.3390/ijerph16214144

McMullen, J. M., George, M., Ingman, B. C., Kuhn, A. P., Graham, D. J., & Carson, R. L. (2020). A systematic review of community engagement outcomes research in school-based health interventions. *Journal of School Health*, *90*(12), 985–994. https://doi.org/10.1111/josh.12962

Medicaid Innovation Accelerator Program. (2019). Medicaid innovation accelerator program state Medicaid-housing agency partnerships toolkit. https://www.medicaid.gov/state-resource-center/innovation-accelerator-program/iap-downloads/functional-areas/mhap-toolkit.pdf

Naleppa, M. J., & Waldbillig, A. A. (2018). International staff exchange: evaluation of a collaborative learning partnership. *International Social Work*, *61*(6), 891–903. https://doi.org/10.1177/0020872816681658

National Academies of Sciences, Engineering, and Medicine. (2021). *The future of nursing 2020–2030: Charting a path to achieve health equity*. The National Academies Press.

National Institute of Nursing Research. (2022). *National institute of nursing research 2022–2026 strategic plan*. https://www.ninr.nih.gov/aboutninr/ninr-mission-and-strategic-plan

Page, J., Kowlowitz, V., & Alden, K. (2010). Development of a scripted unfolding case study focusing on delirium in older adults. *Journal of Continuing Nursing Education*, *41*(5), 225–240. https://doi.org/10.3928/00220124-20100423-05

Potts-Datema, W., Smith, B. J., Taras, H., Lewallen, T. C., Bogden, J. F., & Murray, S. (2005). Successful strategies and lessons learned from development of large-scale partnerships of national non-governmental organizations. *Promotion & Education*, *3*, 131–137.

Protecting youth mental health: The U.S. surgeon general's advisory. (2021). U.S. department of health and human services. https://www.hhs.gov/sites/default/files/surgeon-general-youth-mental-health-advisory.pdf

Rand. (2017). *Evaluation of housing for health permanent supportive housing program*. Hunter, Harvey, Briscombe & Cefalu.

Sacramento County. (2023). Board approves $1.7M to keep homeless housing. *Sac-County News*. https://www.saccounty.gov/news/latest-news/Pages/Board-Approves-1.7-Million-to-Retain-Housing.aspx

Sacramento County. (2019). County-wide collaborative flexible housing pool. *SacCounty News*. https://www.sac-county.gov/news/latest-news/Pages/

County-wide-Collaborative-Flexible-Housing-Pool.aspx

Sauder, K. A., Dabelea, D., Bailey-Callahan, R., Lambert, S. K., Powell, J., James, R., Percy, C., Jenks, B. F., Testaverde, L., Thomas, J. M., Barber, R., Smiley, J., Hockett, C. W., Zhong, V. W., Letourneau, L., Moore, K., Delamater, A. M., & Mayer-Davis, E. (2017). Targeting risk factors for type 2 diabetes in American Indian youth: The tribal turning point pilot study. *Pediatric Obesity*, *13*, 321–329. https://doi.org/10.1111/ijpo.12223

Snyder, J. E., Upton, R. D., Hassett, T. C., Hyunjung, L., Nouri, Z., & Dill, M. (2023). Black representation in the Primary Care Physician workforce and its association with population life expectancy and mortality rates in the US. *JAMA Network Open*, *6*(4), 1–14. https://doi.org/10.1001/jamanetworkopen.2023.6687

Tanner, A., & Stanislo, K. (2022). School nursing research and research implementation priorities. *The Journal of School Nursing*, *38*(6), 500–501. https://doi.org/10.1177/10598405221123231

United Nations Department of Economic and Social Affairs: Disability (n.d.). *List of Non-Governmental Organizations Accredited to the Conference of States Parties*. https://www.un.org/development/desa/disabilities/conference-of-states-parties-to-the-convention-on-the-rights-of-persons-with-disabilities-2/list-of-non-governmental-organization-accredited-to-the-conference-of-states-parties.html

United States Department of Labor. (2022). *DOL Nursing Expansion Grant Program: total funding available: up to $80 million*. https://www.dol.gov/sites/dolgov/files/general/grants/nursing-foa-outreach-flyer.pdf

United States Interagency Council on Homelessness (USICH). (2015). *Opening doors. federal strategic plan to prevent and end homelessness*. USICH.

United States Interagency Council on Homelessness (USICH). (n.d.) https://www.usich.gov/about/usich

Warne, D., & Wescott, S. (2019). Social determinants of American Indian nutritional health. *Current Developments in Nutrition*, *3*(Suppl 2), 12–18. https://doi.org/10.1093/cdn/nzz054

Warren, R. C., Behar-Horenstein, L. S., & Heard, T. V. (2019). Individual perspectives of majority/minority partnerships: Who really benefits and how? *Journal of Health Care for the Poor & Underserved*, *30*(1), 102–115. https://doi.org/10.1353/hpu.2019.0010

Willis, C. D., Corrigan, C., Stockton, L., Greene, J. K., & Riley, B. L. (2017). Exploring the unanticipated effects of multi-sectoral partnerships in chronic disease prevention. *Health Policy*, *121*(2), 158–168. https://doi.org/10.1016/j.healthpol.2016.11.019

World Health Organization., (2023). https://www.who.int/europe/about-us/partnerships/partners/global-health-partnerships

4

Dissemination and Research

Claire McKinley Yoder, PhD, RN, CNE

Jannyse Tapp, DNP, FNP-BC

INTRODUCTION

This chapter emphasizes the influence of research and its dissemination in achieving health equity goals through addressing social and structural determinants of health (SSDH). The Roundtable on Population Health Improvement (2017) underlines the important role of framing research not only in terms of *who* and *what* it studies, but also *why* it does so. This expanded perspective is vital for shifting public thinking regarding health equity and the impact of racism, both a social and structural determinant, on health. Without it, the authors suggest that the public may "rationalize [research findings] away...unless provided powerful cues for how to interpret them" (p. 39). Further complicating the issue are common mental models that resort to euphemisms, steering clear of uncomfortable terms such as *structural racism*. These models often seek middle-ground explanations that obscure the actual causes of inequities, leading to distractions from the essential work of institutional change. There is also a widespread reluctance to openly acknowledge racism and oppression and a hesitance to examine one's own implicit biases (Shahram, 2023). In a systematic review of public health literature from 2002 to 2015, Hardeman et al. (2018) found that although many articles explored institutionalized racism, there was a significant reluctance to mention it in titles or abstracts. They underscore the importance of funding agencies, the review process, and journals in supporting authors to openly acknowledge institutionalized racism as a foundational driver of health inequities. Williams et al. (2019) have issued a clear call for research on racism and health as a fundamental step toward achieving health equity.

Values and Alignment

The NLN-Walden University College of Nursing Institute for Social Determinants of Health and Social Change Leadership Academy underscores the significance of engaging in research and disseminating findings to augment the existing body of evidence pertaining to social and structural determinants of health (SSDH). This commitment to research is rooted in the understanding that a comprehensive understanding of SSDH, their impacts, and potential interventions is crucial for advancing health equity.

By advocating for research conducted from diverse disciplines and by investigators with varying lived experiences, the academy recognizes the multidimensional nature of SSDH. Different perspectives and methodologies contribute to a more holistic understanding of the complex interplay between social determinants and health outcomes. This interdisciplinary approach is essential for developing comprehensive and effective strategies to address health disparities.

The academy's emphasis on diversity is not limited to disciplinary boundaries but extends to geographical, cultural, and other identity factors. This diversity enriches the research and learning experiences of participants, fostering a more comprehensive and nuanced understanding of SSDH. The intersectionality of geographical, disciplinary, and personal identities introduces a breadth of perspectives, enabling participants to appreciate the complexity of social determinants and their varied impacts on health.

Chapter Objectives

Upon completion of this chapter, the learner will be able to:

1. Identify the hallmarks of effective programs to diversify the biomedical workforce.
2. State the importance of a diverse biomedical workforce to the achievement of health equity.
3. Examine disparities in the dissemination of research about racism in nursing publications and analyze their potential implications for advancing health equity.
4. Explore the historical context of racism and discriminatory practices in the nursing profession.

CONSIDERATIONS AND BACKGROUND

Several barriers to this research include the position of the researcher in the research process, the increased workload and lack of mentorship of academic researchers from historically excluded and underrepresented identities, and challenges with dissemination of results through publishing. Evidence of the trends impacting research and dissemination on racism and health equity are provided in two exemplars later in this chapter:

▸ Exemplar 1: A scoping review of the research on diversity in the biomedical research workforce and programs to increase diversity in this field

▸ Exemplar 2: A bibliometric analysis of the scholarly literature in nursing on racism

The researcher's characteristics—including gender, racial identity, and socioeconomic status—exert a substantial influence on their research endeavors (Coghlan & Brydon-Miller, 2014). These characteristics impact not only the research questions posed but also the study's design, execution, interpretation, and outcomes (Coghlan & Brydon-Miller, 2014; Olukotun et al., 2021). Furthermore, researcher traits have ramifications for research funding. Hoppe et al. (2019) discovered that 20% of the funding disparity in National Institutes of Health R01 awards between Black and White researchers was attributable to their chosen research topics.

Historically, the scholarly knowledge related to non-White groups is limited in health (Zambrana & Williams, 2022), with more available about Black populations and much less related to Indigenous groups. By the 1970s and 1980s, because of improvements in access to higher education for underrepresented groups, there was an increase in professionals and researchers from underrepresented identities (Zambrana & Williams, 2022). Despite this, significant inequities in the number of individuals from underrepresented backgrounds continue in health and health research fields. This has multiple effects, including biases in education, research, funding, and dissemination of research (Holmes, 2020; Shahram, 2023; Zambrana & Williams, 2022).

Another barrier to conducting and disseminating research by academic researchers from underrepresented communities is that they face a "cultural tax" or "minority tax," which results in increased workload and less time to devote to scholarship and teaching (Faucett et al., 2022; Guillaume & Apodaca, 2022). As a smaller proportion of the academy, faculty of color are disproportionately asked to take on additional service activities, such as advising and mentoring students of color, committee work, and education of other faculty on diversity issues (Guillaume & Apodaca, 2022). These additional responsibilities—which are often not considered as highly in the promotion and tenure process—may keep diverse faculty from research and dissemination endeavors, thus blocking their attainment of promotion and tenure (Amaechi et al., 2021).

SOLUTIONS AND CHANGING APPROACH

One way to address this barrier is through mentoring programs to help early career faculty negotiate the many competing demands for their time and to support their leadership development (Hamilton & Haozous, 2017). The first exemplar in this chapter discusses the current status of diversity in the biomedical research workforce and explores ways to increase it. A notable finding is that mentoring is a hallmark of most of these programs. With the limited number of experienced researchers that can serve as mentors, it is essential to maximize their reach. Julion et al. (2019) suggest a novel hybrid peer mentoring method to address the limited number of senior faculty that can serve as mentors. Identifying creative methods to sustain mentorship for diverse students and early career researchers without overwhelming the few mid- and later-stage researchers is critical to increasing the diversity of the biomedical research workforce.

EXEMPLAR 1: REVIEW OF LITERATURE ON DIVERSITY IN THE BIOMEDICAL WORKFORCE

A scoping review was conducted to answer two questions:

1. What is the scope of scholarly research about diversity in health research workforce development? Specifically, what research has been done to identify the state of diversity in the health and biomedical research workforce?
2. What is the scope of programs to diversify the future researcher workforce?

Methods

This scoping review adhered to the methodology outlined by Arksey and O'Malley (2005). The choice of a scoping review was driven by the aim of summarizing the existing research pertaining to the development of a diverse research workforce in health and biomedical research, along with literature focused on programs designed to enhance workforce diversity. The search terms "research" and "workforce" were combined with "nurs*," "med*," or "health*," and "diversity," or "equity." Searches were conducted in databases including CINAHL Plus with Full Text, ERIC, Health Source, Nursing/Academic Edition, and Medline. To retrieve the most pertinent publications, the results were narrowed down to peer-reviewed literature published between January 1, 2013, and June 31, 2023.

The inclusion criteria comprised: 1) completed research studies pertaining to diversity in the research workforce or workforce development programs; or 2) descriptions of programs designed to enhance diversity in the health-related and biomedical research workforce. Exclusion criteria were applied to publications that centered on faculty not identified as researchers, abstract-only documents, and study protocols. Data from selected publications were extracted into an Excel database developed by the researchers, building on the framework employed in previous literature reviews and tailored to the specific requirements of the current review.

Results

The search initially yielded 162 publications, with 44 meeting the inclusion criteria (see Figure 4.1). The broadness of the search terms likely contributed to a substantial number of irrelevant documents. Through citation searching of the included studies, an additional 26 articles that met the inclusion criteria were discovered. Of the 70 articles included in the review, 24 were program descriptions (refer to Table 4.1), and 46 were

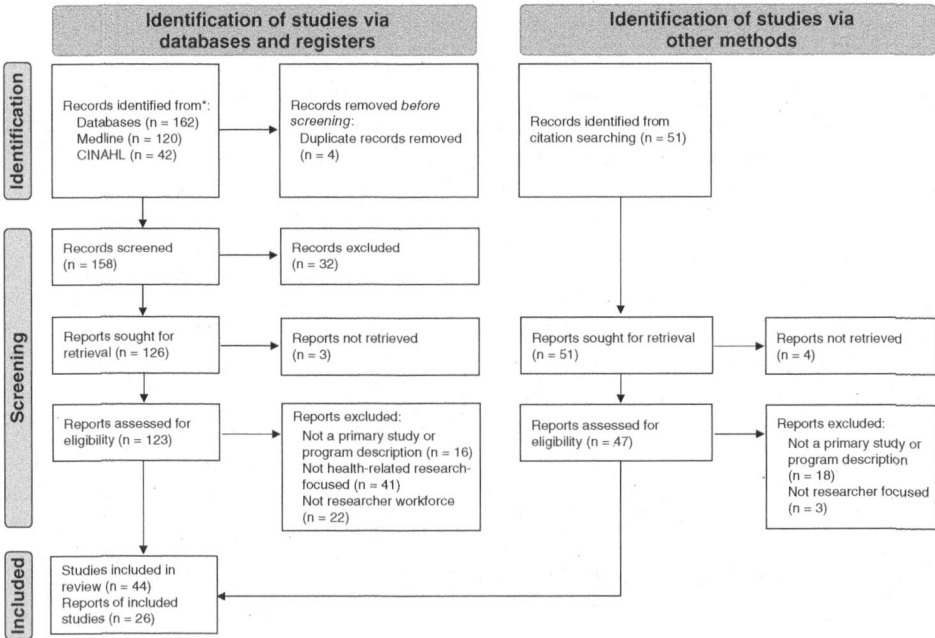

FIGURE 4.1 PRISMA diagram. (Source: Page, M. J., McKenzie, J. E., Bossuyt, P. M., Boutron, I., Hoffmann, T. C., Mulrow, C. D., et al. The PRISMA 2020 statement: an updated guideline for reporting systematic reviews. *BMJ* 2021;372:n71. doi: 10.1136/bmj.n71. For more information, visit: http://www.prisma-statement.org/)

TABLE 4.1

Program Descriptions*

Author/Program	Level	Mentoring	Research Experience	Length	Other	Outcomes (If Provided)
Abebe et al., 2019; Rubio et al., 2018; CEED	EC	Yes	No	1 year	Coursework, monthly seminars, networking, training in scientific and grant writing, research presentation, and other skills	45 grads: 76% female, 78% non-White. Increased publications. Increased likelihood to be an assistant professor
Boyington et al., 2016; PRIDE	EC	Yes, over 2 years	Yes	Two 2–3-week summer sessions	Grant writing support, special lectures, workshops, and courses in research-specific areas	n/a
Brandon et al., 2014; Bridge to Doctorate	G	Yes	Yes	2+ years	Research courses, enhancement experiences	n/a
Butler et al., 2017; HELI	PD/EC	No	No	5 days	Research specific sessions, funding, leadership development	73% of participants promoted, 23% secured independent federal funding
Canner et al., 2017; BD2K	UG	Yes	Yes, varies	Varies	Varies depending on program	n/a
Crockett, 2014; REPID	UG/G	Yes	Yes	1 year	Basics of research education, personal and professional development; funding for research presentation	In the program's first 3 years, 51 students joined, with 36 completing research training, and 80% continued research afterward.

(continued)

TABLE 4.1

Program Descriptions* (Continued)

Author/Program	Level	Mentoring	Research Experience	Length	Other	Outcomes (If Provided)
Croff et al., 2022; HBRN	UG/G	Yes	Yes	Varies	Attending and presenting at HBRN calls and national conferences	70% alumni engaged in research or education, 2 publications, and 20 conference presentations
Crump et al., 2015; Summer Residential Program (SRP)	HS	Yes	Yes	5 weeks	Inquiry-based curriculum	SRP participants (54/54) entered college, surpassing comparisons, and doubling the statewide average, showcasing strong matching in the groups.
Duffus et al., 2014; Imhotep	UG	No	Yes	11-week summer program	Intensive 2-week coursework	All 481 trained students earned bachelor's degrees. 73.2% pursued further education, 53% master's, 11.1% medical, and 7.3% other doctoral degrees. 60% entered public health careers.
Estape et al., 2018; RCMI programs at University of Puerto Rico and Morehouse School of Medicine	G, EC	Yes, monthly	Yes	2-4 years	Focused recruitment, scholar incentives, awards to cover research expenses and travel, salary support, and career development	Results: >50% women, all BIPOC scholars, MDs and PhDs largest disciplines, varied representation. Graduates secured 74% funding (23% NIH)
Fernandez et al., 2016; HPTN, RAMP, ATN, and SBSRN	G, EC	Yes, all	Yes	HPTN: 18 months RAMP: 2-4 months or 9–12 months ATN: 36 months SBSRN: unclear	HPTN: additional professional/career development; ATN: research development aligned with ATN's research agenda	HPTN: 5 years, 11 publications, 7 presentations. RAMP: 38 scholars over 4 years, increased HIV vaccine research interest. ATN: 6 scholars, all first-author manuscripts. SBSRN: 79 interdisciplinary HIV researchers

Fuchs et al., 2016; SHARP–Summer HIV/AIDS Research Program (SHARP) at the San Francisco Department of Public Health	UG	Yes	12-week	Didactic seminars for content and research methods, and networking opportunities	From 2012 to 2015, SHARP's initial four cohorts developed research skills, grew in self-confidence as scientists, and most alumni now work in research positions or are pursuing graduate studies related to HIV prevention. All SHARP scholars have completed the program, and when eligible, attained their college degrees.
Gandhi et al., 2014; Ghandhi & Johnson, 2016; Johnson & Gandhi, 2014; Mentoring the Mentors	MLC	Workshop to develop mentoring abilities	2-day training for mid- or later-stage investigators to gain mentoring skills for researchers from underrepresented groups	Workshops covered mentoring techniques and diversity-related topics, including unconscious bias, microaggressions, description of diversity supplements in grants, resiliency, and self-awareness.	In HIV research, multiple disciplines were involved. Professors made up 51%; Associate Professors 37%; and senior Assistant Professors 11%. Most (66%) mentored 1–3 mentees; 33% mentored 4 or more. Training domains included communication, leadership, mentoring tools, productivity, diversity, time management, funding, literature, and life-work balance.
Howell et al., 2019; Edmonson Internship	UG	Yes	8-week summer internship	Basic research skills and training (including compliance training), which are chiefly fulfilled online prior to joining the program. Didactic lectures in various domains; tours and shadowing experiences.	93% agreed Edmondson internship was important for their career development. 46/48 who applied for opportunities found it advantageous. Many pursued further education or training.

(continued)

TABLE 4.1

Program Descriptions* (Continued)

Author/Program	Level	Mentoring	Research Experience	Length	Other	Outcomes (If Provided)
Huerta et al., 2022; Marriot et al., 2022; Marriott et al., 2021; Knight Scholars	HS	Yes, peer mentors and research mentors	Yes, in year 2 and in year 3	3 years, summer 1 is 1 week, summer 3 is 10 weeks	The Knight Scholars Program is a tiered program that increases in duration and intensity over a 3-year period.	70% of Knight Scholars were female, 15% reported disability, 77% reported a disadvantaged background, and 32% were multilingual. Peer mentors reported growth in professional communication (82%), wanted to continue biomedical sciences (100%), mentoring (100%), and increased interest in cancer (73%).
Jean-Louis et al., 2016; NYU PRIDE Institute	EC	Yes, throughout 2-year program	No	Summer 1: 2-week didactic program Summer 2: 1-week NIH proposal-focused program	Other activities include mid-year meetings, monthly webinars, and Summer 1 workshops on research conduct, biostatistics, grant writing, and sleep medicine.	PRIDE scholars' NIH award success rate (33%) surpasses contemporaneous investigators (17.4%). All aim for health disparities research careers, 85% in sleep health disparities research. Challenges include academic workload, isolation as faculty from underrepresented groups, and a sense of racial isolation.

Jones et al., 2020; IMSD Program	UG/G	Multi-tiered mentoring approach: major advisor, peer mentoring, and coaching	No	2 years	Trainees get financial support, personalized development plans, culturally aware research experiences, and professional development. There's also a prematriculation summer program.	56% female, 54% African American/Black, 40% Hispanic/Latino, 61% from *institutions of higher education that serve underrepresented groups.* 40%–74% of trainees earned their PhD (cohort 1 and 2)
López et al., 2021; Pathmaker Program	HS	Yes, student and research mentors	Yes	12 weeks	Lab-intensive training course, HIPAA, and CITI training. Professional development activities.	PathMaker trainees are more diverse than the university population: Black (+15%), Latinx (+29%), AI/AN (+6%), Asian (+26%), and female (+22%) representation. 77% of alumni declared STEM majors. They secured NCI research funding and participated in prestigious research programs. Of 43 alumni, 32 were in undergrad programs, 11 have graduated: 5 had STEM jobs, 1 was in a STEM PhD program, 2 were in medical school, and 3 were lost to follow-up. All incoming high school seniors have completed high school and are now in college.

(*continued*)

TABLE 4.1

Program Descriptions* (Continued)

Author/Program	Level	Mentoring	Research Experience	Length	Other	Outcomes (If Provided)
Norris et al., 2020; NIH BUILD programs at 10 universities	UG	Not provided	Not provided	Not provided	Not provided	Of student participants: 65% female, mean age 18.5 ± 1.9 years (range: 15–64). Racial composition: 18% Hispanic/Latinx, 19% African American/Black, 2% Native Hawaiian/Pacific Islander or American Indian/Alaska Native, 17% Asian, 29% White, 14% reported two or more races. 27% had income <$30,000/year, 25% first-generation in college, and 28% reported a disability. Outcomes were not included.
Ofili et al., 2019; RCMI Program	EC, MLC	Yes, coaching and mentoring program	Yes	Varies	Scholars joined grant writing program, collaborated to develop concepts into research projects, and competed for pilot research awards.	Increased collaboration with more coauthored manuscripts; RCMI program contributed significantly to doctoral degrees for AA and Hispanics in 2002 and 2012; RCMI RTRN supported NRMN to recruit diverse early-stage investigators.
Richardson et al., 2017; BUILD EXITO	UG	Career and peer mentoring	Yes	Varies	Orientation, career mentor and peer mentor, enrichment workshops, basic research foundations gateway course, and research mentor match	n/a

Rivers et al., 2020; HS-STEP-UP	HS	Research mentor	Yes	8–10 weeks during summer	RCR training, research team skills, CITI training, webinars, NIH conference, and college prep workshops were part of the program.	193 students: 82% underrepresented groups, 23% first-gen college, 67% female, diverse racial backgrounds, 48% <$37,000/year income, and all attended college.
Rubio et al., 2018; PROMISED; LEADS; ENACT; TL1	G, PD, EC	Professional Mentoring Skills Enhancing Diversity (PROMISED) program. LEADS: no ENACT: no TL1: mentored research	PROMISED program: no LEADS: no ENACT: no TL1: yes	Varies	Varies by program—provides professional research development skills training	CEED I and II trained 76 URB scholars in 10 years. TL1 had 17% from URBs, PROMISED had 39% from underrepresented backgrounds. 58 participants across 2 years, 21 in Career Coaching Workshop and online modules. LEADS trained 42 scholars across three cohorts, starting with four institutions of higher education that serve underrepresented groups. ENACT trained 113 investigators in PCOR methods.
Smalley & Warren, 2020; DESRE	UG, G	Peer mentoring	Yes	6-week, intensive, full-time, residential training program	Didactic courses, community immersion experiences, ethics training	In four summers, DESRE enrolled 22 students (3 predoctoral, 4 masters, 15 undergraduates). Achieved a 77% success rate in promoting careers in biomedical research and health disparity elimination. All participants from underrepresented groups entered graduate programs or health equity careers.

(continued)

TABLE 4.1

Program Descriptions* (Continued)

Author/Program	Level	Mentoring	Research Experience	Length	Other	Outcomes (If Provided)
Sopher et al., 2015; RAMP	G	Yes	Yes	One year	Training workshops, quarterly seminars	RAMP program: Of 13 medical students (62% male) completing RAMP, 54% African American, 46% Hispanic. 54% in year 1–2, 23% year-long projects. The majority (77%) focused on social/behavioral research. 69% domestic, 31% international sites. Pre-post program assessment showed significant knowledge and skill improvements.
Tagge et al., 2021; TRANSCENDS	EC	Year-long mentoring	No	One year	Online MSCR program; monthly webinars; sessions at American Academy of Neurology meeting	n/a
Thorpe et al., 2020; NRMN STAR	EC	No	No	12 months	Grantsmanship training	STAR trainees improved grant writing self-efficacy. 62% Black, 62% female, 90% had PhDs. 24% lacked postdoctoral training; 29% worked at institutions of higher education that serve underrepresented groups.

Urizar et al., 2017	UG	Yes	Yes	Varies	Learning community, courses in research methods, communications, CITI training, GRE prep, research colloquia	n/a
Vishwanatha et al., 2019; TABS	HS, UG, G, PD, EC	Varies	Varies	Varies		Collaborative programs with schools reached 7,500+ students. Trained 1,166 students and faculty, produced 130 manuscripts. Past fellows, advanced careers.
Williams et al., 2016; The Academy	G	Career mentors	No	One year	Group career coaching	Baseline data showed female students and students from underrepresented groups had similar academic career perceptions. Academy students significantly improved their perceptions.
Zhou et al., 2021; PASS	UG	Weekly mentor meetings	Yes	8 weeks each summer over 2 years	Didactic courses, community observation experiences, book club discussions.	Respondents' self-reported competence in their ability to do research increased significantly after summer of PASS. Participants noted mentoring was especially helpful.

HS, high school students; UG, undergraduate students; G, graduate students; PD, postdoctoral; EC, early career researcher; MLC, mid- or late-career researcher. ATN, Adolescent Trials Network for HIV/AIDS Interventions; CEED, Career Education and Enhancement for Health Care Diversity; CITI, Collaborative Institutional Training Initiative; ENACT, Expanding National Capacity in PCOR Through Training; HBRN, Healthy Brain Research Network; HIPPA, The Health Insurance Portability and Accountability Act; HPTN, HIV Prevention Trials Network; IMSD, Initiative for Maximizing Student Development; LEADS, Leading Emerging and Diverse Scientists to Success; MSCR, Master of Science in Clinical Research; PASS, Penn Access Summer Scholars; PCOR, Patient-Centered Outcomes Research; RAMP, Research and Mentoring Program; RCR, Responsible Conduct of Research; SBSRN, Social and Behavioral Science Research Network; STAR, Steps Toward Academic Research.

*Note: In this table, the word "male" refers to a person assigned male at birth, and the word "female" refers to a person assigned female at birth.

research articles (refer to Table 4.2). Among the research-based articles, 33 were evaluations of programs aimed at fostering diversity in health and biomedical research initiatives. Eleven articles assessed specific National Institutes of Health (NIH) grant awards, including seven studies on diversity in NIH R01 awards, and one each on K awards, NINR, T-32, and NIH-funded workforce programs. Notably, all studies and programs were conducted within the United States. Additionally, 45 percent ($n = 32$) of the articles in this review had at least one author affiliated with an institution of higher education serving underrepresented groups.

The included studies covered various study areas, including biomedical science (25), health care-related topics (e.g., health services, health disparities) (15), HIV-related research (6), behavioral studies (4), pediatrics (3), clinical and translational research (3), cancer (2), biomedical data science (2), rehabilitation (2), nursing (2), MD-PhD researchers (2), gerontology (2), medicine (2), and single studies in rehabilitation, public health, neurology, head and neck surgery, pathology and laboratory medicine, precision medicine, and sleep (some documents encompassed more than one study area). These programs primarily targeted early-career researchers (13) and graduate students (13), followed by undergraduates (12), postdoctoral level researchers (8), high school students (6), and mid- to late-career investigators (4). For a detailed breakdown, refer to Table 4.3, which illustrates the patterns identified within the literature based on the Patterns, Advances, Gaps, Evidence for Practice and Research (PAGER) Framework (Bradbury-Jones et al., 2022).

Discussion

Although there is a clear appreciation for the importance of nurturing a diverse workforce in the health and biomedical sciences, the existing infrastructure appears to prioritize graduate programs for early-stage investigators. There is a lack of programs targeting high schools, and only one program was identified for grades K-8. Notably, Hoff et al. (2022) emphasized that adolescents' career interests are closely connected to eventual career choices. Therefore, initiatives aimed at adolescents could be instrumental in expanding the pipeline of diverse biomedical researchers.

It is noteworthy that in most of the research included in this study, diversity was often limited to binary categories such as gender and racial/ethnic groups. However, some research studies did consider a broader range of factors, including disability, disadvantaged background, age, being the first generation in a family to attend college, low-income status, educational disadvantages, citizenship status, country of birth or citizenship, sexual orientation, urban/rural background, and personal adversity. Taking an intersectional approach, which considers these multiple dimensions of diversity, provides a more comprehensive understanding and a richer set of personal experiences. Researchers who view their work through an intersectional lens can formulate more contextually relevant research questions, conduct more nuanced studies, engage in more meaningful partnerships with diverse communities, and draw more comprehensive conclusions from their research. This broader perspective on diversity is essential for achieving equity in research.

Furthermore, it is important to create more opportunities for students from diverse backgrounds to explore research careers. This can begin in schools by exposing children to research-related professions, extending through adolescence with opportunities

TABLE 4.2

Research Studies*

Author(s), Year	Research Area	Type of Article	Study Aim(s)/Hypotheses	Outcomes	Level of Participants
Abebe et al., 2019	Health care	Evaluation study of program.	Quantify program effectiveness of the CEED program.	45 grads, 76% female, 78% non-White. Increased publications, increased likelihood to be Assistant Professor	EC
Andriole & Jeffe, 2016	MD-PhD graduates	National cohort analysis.	Examine the extent to which recent MD-PhD program graduates received full-time academic medicine faculty appointments.	Graduates from schools with MSTP funding and >1 year of residency research were more likely to secure faculty appointments. However, Asian/Pacific Islander and graduates from underrepresented groups, those with >$100,000 in debt, and those in surgical and other specialties were less likely. Gender didn't significantly impact faculty appointments.	D
Andriole et al., 2017	Health-related research	Quantitative descriptive study of mentored K-awards.	As candidate review criteria for mentored K awards include consideration of an applicant's research experiences and academic record.	Graduates from underrepresented groups received fewer K awards. Graduates who were not from underrepresented groups were more likely to have participated in research electives, earned authorship, and graduated from MD-PhD programs. Additionally, such graduates were more likely to complete ≥1 GME-research year and receive F32 awards. The study suggests that promoting student participation in productive research activities during and after medical school for those in underrepresented groups could reduce racial/ethnic disparities in K award receipt.	PD/ED

(continued)

69

TABLE 4.2

Research Studies* (Continued)

Author(s), Year	Research Area	Type of Article	Study Aim(s)/Hypotheses	Outcomes	Level of Participants
Awad et al., 2022	Biomedical data science	Cross-sectional survey	Summarize NIMHD-funded RCMI institutions' efforts for data science training programs.	RCMI-funded institutions had BIPOC student majorities (80%–100%) with varying male-to-female ratios (62/38 to 40/60). Research encompassed Basic (37%), Clinical Translational (32%), and Social/Behavioral (32%) domains. Most programs focused on graduate students, faculty from Instructors to Full Professors, and Post-Docs/Fellows; only one targeted undergraduates. Challenges included data access, external faculty recruitment, and scheduling. Recommendations for diversity improvement comprised diverse data sets, training across learner levels and underrepresented groups, infrastructure enhancement, sustainable funding, and diverse faculty recruitment.	UG/G
Brenner et al., 2022	Otolaryngology, head and neck surgery	Evaluation	To what extent does CORE engender diversity, equity, and inclusion in otolaryngology?	Distribution of awards was somewhat equitable; otolaryngology has a significant lack of diversity. Some years there were no grant recipients of color. Women are more successful in securing this grant funding. Most grant recipients were in a small number of residency programs.	EC, MLC

| Croff et al., 2022 | Gerontological, Aging, Cognitive Health Research | Mixed methods program evaluation of CDC Healthy Brain Research Network Scholars Program (HBRN) | Evaluation of HBRN Program. | Most HBRN Scholars (75.6%) were female. The group was diverse, including non-Latino White people (39.0%), African American people (19.5%), Asian people (14.6%), and Hispanics/Latino people (14.6%). They primarily came from graduate programs, with some undergraduates and postdoctoral students. Affiliations spanned Medicine, Public Health, Nursing, Social Work, and other fields. Afterward, 70.0% secured positions such as program coordinators, research assistants, postdoctoral fellows, or assistant professors. They collectively produced 2 publications and 20 conference presentations. Alumni cited increased research experience, networking, mentorship, and knowledge of HBRN projects as benefits from the program. | UG/G |
| Crump et al., 2015 | Biomedical science | Comparative study and description of Summer Research Program (SRP) | Describe preliminary results after 4 years of follow-up. | The SRP participants and the comparison group were closely matched in terms of various factors. All SRP participants (54/54) enrolled in college, surpassing both the comparison group and the statewide average. A similar proportion of both groups aimed to major in biological sciences or health-related fields ($p = .82$). In essence, SRP attracted high-achieving applicants who achieved notably better educational outcomes than the general population. | HS |

TABLE 4.2

Research Studies* (Continued)

Author(s), Year	Research Area	Type of Article	Study Aim(s)/Hypotheses	Outcomes	Level of Participants
Doyle et al., 2021	Physician-scientists vs biomedical researchers	Mixed methods study of the effects of COVID-19 pandemic on early career physician-scientists	Compare the impact of COVID-19 on the lives of 196 early-career physician-scientists vs. PhD researchers who are underrepresented in biomedical research.	Both physician-scientists and PhD researchers experienced disruptions to work, difficulties concentrating, and increased overall stress during the pandemic. However, more PhD researchers reported increased productivity, schedule flexibility, and quality time with family compared to physician-scientists. Physician-scientists faced challenges due to increased clinical demands and the risk of exposing family members to the virus, leading to psychological distress and family strain since the pandemic began.	EC
Duffus et al., 2014	Public health sciences	Quantitative descriptive study of Imhotep program	To describe the Imhotep program and highlight some of its outcomes.	100% of the 481 trained students earned bachelor's degrees; 73.2% earned graduate degrees (53% earned master's degrees, 11.1% earned medical degrees, and 7.3% earned other doctoral degrees); and 60% entered public health careers.	UG

					PD/EC
Duncan et al., 2016	Biomedical science	Qualitative study	Assess the effectiveness of the current NHLBI diversity program, improve strategies toward achieving its goal, and provide guidance for the transition of recipients' grant support.	Diverse trainees faced several key issues, including the cost of living, family planning, exposure to science at a young age, retention of faculty from underrepresented groups, career exploration, research limitations during postdocs, securing funding, and finding external mentors. Proposed support mechanisms encompass adjusting stipends for living costs, loan repayment aid, family support, childcare assistance for postdocs, parental leave, flexible work hours, science programs for diverse high school students, increased funding for diverse undergraduates, and university accountability in retaining faculty from underrepresented groups.	
Duong et al., 2023	Clinical and Translational Science	Cross-sectional survey	Identify the extent to which CTSA Program members perceived DEI to be important, as well as the extent to which members were committed to improving DEI.	The majority (72.7%) rated DEI as "extremely important." Over half (56.3%) were "extremely committed" to making fundamental CTSA changes. 86.2% were very or extremely committed to DEI improvements. Barriers included funding, institutional/CTSA commitment, and DEI outreach, recruitment, retention, and advancement. PIs and Executive Directors were less committed, emphasizing the need for leadership in driving change.	EC, MLC
Erosheva et al., 2020	Health-related research	Quantitative research study	Evaluate whether racial disparities in impact scores can be explained by application and applicant characteristics.	Preliminary scores account for racial disparities but not all score variability. From 2014 to 2016, R01 applications from Black individuals had a 55% lower award rate than those from White individuals (10.2% vs. 18.5%), resulting in a 45% funding gap. Matched applications with similar characteristics had award rates of 11.57% for Black and 15.39% for White applicants.	EC, MLC

(continued)

TABLE 4.2

Research Studies* (*Continued*)

Author(s), Year	Research Area	Type of Article	Study Aim(s)/Hypotheses	Outcomes	Level of Participants
Fernandez et al., 2021	Health Sciences	Qualitative study	Investigate the viewpoint of female early-stage investigators (within 10 years of their terminal degree and without substantial NIH research grants).	To diversify health sciences, acknowledge and accommodate family responsibilities. Female leaders benefit early-career women. Inequities in faculty work distribution exist. Address gender equity in committees, service, and administrative tasks. Recognize and reward women's multiple roles inside and outside work. Accommodate these roles in career progression expectations.	EC
Flores et al., 2016	Pediatrics	Thematic analysis of conference discussion.	Identify urgent priorities and how to ensure success for young investigators from underrepresented racial/ethnic groups.	Six topics identified by young investigators: negotiating for research time, adapting to changing academic career paths, incorporating nonacademic work, addressing racism and discrimination, handling isolation as faculty from underrepresented groups, and improving mentoring for future academics.	EC
Flores et al., 2019	Pediatrics	Delphi Research Study	Provide a guide to academic success for young investigators from underrepresented groups.	Most important factors for success: Mentorship, consistent writing, securing research time, passion for the subject, proper training, persistence, and learning from failures.	EC

Forscher et al., 2019	Health-related research	Quantitative research study	Identifying if PI names associated with being a White person or a Black person, male or female affects NIH R01 reviews.	The study found no evidence of different overall impact scores based on the PI's race or gender. Proposals with White male PIs were evaluated similarly to those with White female, Black male, or Black female PIs, regardless of proposal quality, topic, or reviewer's identity.	EC, MLC
Frogner, 2018	Health services research	Quantitative exploratory descriptive analysis	Describe the stock and supply of Health Service Researchers (HSR) in the United States.	Between 2007 and 2015, the stock of HSRs increased by about 3,000, or 25 percent. However, the educational pipeline has slowed in recent years, with doctoral degrees in core HSR fields remaining flat or declining. About half of master's and doctoral degree recipients were non-White or Hispanic, with Black/African Americans being prominent. Hispanic representation was comparatively lower than in the general population. White, non-Hispanics increased their doctoral degree representation by 10.7 percentage points, and Black/African Americans by 4.3 percentage points.	PD
Frogner, 2022	Health services research (HSR)	Quantitative research study	Identify the size and diversity of the current HSR workforce and recent graduates from HSR-related programs.	The number of master's and doctoral graduates from core fields has increased consistently. Females are well represented among recent graduates compared to the US population. Academy Health's membership is more racially diverse, with higher Asian representation, but lower Black/African American and Hispanic representation. However, Black/African American and Hispanic graduates in core HSR fields have been increasing, offering potential for closing these gaps with focused efforts.	G, EC, MLC

(continued)

TABLE 4.2

Research Studies* (Continued)

Author(s), Year	Research Area	Type of Article	Study Aim(s)/Hypotheses	Outcomes	Level of Participants
Ghaffarzadegan et al., 2014	Biomedical science	Simulation-based analyses of effects of different policies	Understand the dynamics of change in the number of national and international Postdocs (PDs).	Mapping postdoctoral careers may favor foreign postdocs and reduce the ratio of national to international postdocs in the USA. Diversity in the research workforce is influenced more by K–graduate education policies than postgraduate ones.	PD
Ghaffarzadegan et al., 2015	Biomedical science	Quantitative research study	Analyze the number of PhD graduates in biomedical areas and identify whether there is overproduction of PhDs.	The scarcity of tenure-track positions (1 for every 6.3 PhD graduates) leads to underemployment for many PhDs, who may work in lower-paid positions or outside academia. Universities benefit from this skilled, low-cost workforce, reinforcing the cycle. Postdocs enable faculty to handle more research, driving the growth of new PhDs, especially in industry and research centers.	D
Gibbs et al., 2014	Biomedical science	Quantitative research study	Are there distinct career interest patterns based on social identity (race/ethnicity, gender, and their intersection) in recent BMS Ph.D. graduates?	Women from underrepresented groups reported lower interest in faculty careers at research universities compared to well-represented females and other social-identity groups. This pattern was specific to this career path and not seen in all faculty careers or research-based careers. Factors like publication record and advisor support positively influenced interest, while obtaining a PhD from a Top 50 university had a negative impact.	D

Source	Topic	Type	Purpose	Findings	Themes
Gibbs et al., 2016	Biomedical PhDs in medical school basic science departments	Quantitative research study	Identify changes in the numbers of biomedical PhDs and assistant professorships in medical school basic science departments by scientists from underrepresented groups and well-represented backgrounds between 1980 and 2014.	The study reveals that the increase in the pool of potential assistant professor candidates from underrepresented groups has not significantly influenced the hiring of faculty from underrepresented groups. Despite the growth in the number of people from underrepresented groups earning PhDs, the modeling suggests that assistant professors from underrepresented groups in basic science departments of U.S. medical schools may remain below 10% by 2080, even without discrimination, challenging the pipeline explanation for the lack of faculty members from underrepresented groups.	G, EC
Ginther et al., 2016	Health-related research	Quantitative research study	Analyze the relationship between gender, race/ethnicity, and the probability of being awarded an R01 grant from the National Institutes of Health (NIH).	The majority of applicants were PhD holders, predominantly men and White individuals. Only 5.1% of applications came from women of color. Race had a more significant impact on NIH funding outcomes than gender, with applications from Asian people and Black people being less likely to receive funding compared to White people. Despite controlling for various factors, women PhDs applied for fewer grants and were consequently less likely to receive R01 awards over the studied decades.	EC, MLC

(continued)

TABLE 4.2

Research Studies* (Continued)

Author(s), Year	Research Area	Type of Article	Study Aim(s)/Hypotheses	Outcomes	Level of Participants
Harawa et al., 2017	Gerontological/Aging/Cognitive Health Research	Qualitative evaluation of program	Identify optimal approaches to shaping and assessing mentorship programs for faculty from underrepresented groups in health research careers.	We need to broaden the definition of "success" beyond NIH's emphasis on research productivity and academic positions. Various research products, such as lay publications, presentations, and social media, can contribute to addressing health disparities in aging populations. URM faculty often carry additional responsibilities representing people of color in various settings. RCMAR mentors help mentees manage extracurricular requests, prioritizing scholarship and career advancement. All RCMAR center awards have been granted to research-intensive institutions.	EC/MLC
Heggeness et al., 2016	Health-related research	Quantitative research study	To measure diversity within the National Institutes of Health (NIH)-funded workforce.	In NIH-funded programs, women and under-represented groups are well-represented in training and early career mentored programs but underrepresented in independent research awards. White, Asian, and Hispanic citizens are overrepresented in the independent researcher pool, with almost equal representation for White women. In contrast, Black men and women, Hispanic women, and Asian women are underrepresented. Women of all racial and ethnic groups are less likely to be in the R01-equivalent pool than the RPG awardee pool, while men of all racial and ethnic groups except Black people are more likely to be in the R01-equivalent pool. The RPG awardee pool is more diverse than the R01-equivalent awardee pool.	PD, EC, MLC

Hill et al., 2023	Medicine	Quantitative research study	Analyze diversity supplement utilization by medical schools.	While diversity supplements for R01 grants have grown over the last 15 years, they are still relatively rare among medical schools. Top 40 medical schools are not more likely than others to have diversity supplement funding. This study indicates that many medical schools might be missing chances to mentor and support faculty of color by not actively pursuing diversity supplements.	G
Hoppe et al., 2019	Health-related research	Quantitative research study	To identify underlying causes of funding gap in AA/Black scientists.	Three key factors contribute to the funding gap between African American/Black (AA/B) and White (WH) applicants. AA/B applications are less likely to be discussed during study sections, receive lower impact scores when discussed, and often focus on community and population-level research, accounting for 21% of the funding gap. This contrasts with more fundamental and mechanistic investigations chosen by WH applicants.	EC, MLC
Jean-Louis et al., 2016	Sleep medicine	Mixed methods program evaluation from NYU PRIDE Institute	To evaluate the NIH-funded PRIDE Institute in Behavioral Medicine and Sleep Disorders Research at New York University Langone Medical Center.	PRIDE scholars outperformed their peers in securing NIH awards. However, they faced various challenges, including being the sole faculty members from underrepresented groups, managing clinical and research responsibilities, feeling isolated, and dealing with unspoken racial issues.	EC
Jeske et al., 2022	Precision medicine	Qualitative research study	Identify meanings of and challenges to equitable diversification, precision medicine research (PMR), teams.	Underrepresented individuals are often hired in frontline research staff roles and seen as diversity experts. Existing power structures hinder diverse team growth. Creating mentorship, opportunities, and meaningful inclusion is essential for equity.	EC/MLC

(continued)

TABLE 4.2

Research Studies* (Continued)

Author(s), Year	Research Area	Type of Article	Study Aim(s)/Hypotheses	Outcomes	Level of Participants
Johnson & Gandhi, 2015	HIV Research	Quantitative research study	Measure mentoring competency after a training workshop for HIV researchers interested in mentoring early-stage investigators of diversity.	Mentor training domains were ranked, with communication strategies as the highest. Attendees showed significant improvement in self-rated mentoring skills across six domains, including communication, aligning expectations, assessing understanding, addressing diversity, fostering independence, and promoting professional development.	EC/MLC
Kaatz et al., 2016	Health-related research	Quantitative research study	Authors hypothesized that application priority and criteria scores, and categories of words in critiques, would differ between male and female PIs.	Differences in reviewers' evaluations between male and female principal investigators (PIs) were found, particularly for Type 2 R01 applications. Female PIs applying for Type 2 R01s may face scoring disadvantages, with poorer ratings in priority, approach, and significance. Text analysis revealed potential variations in evaluative standards for male and female PIs in Type 2 applications. Additionally, linguistic distinctions were observed in the strengths' sections of the approach and significance criteria for funded applications.	EC/MLC

Kameny et al., 2014	Behavioral science	Qualitative	Examine barriers to career success for researchers in the behavioral sciences from underrepresented groups.	Participants spanned diverse fields (e.g., social work, psychology, and medicine), with 52% early-career and 48% mid-career. Barriers included institutional factors like promotion policies, mentorship gaps, and departmental politics. Cultural issues related to race (72%) and gender (26%) played a role, with racism and undervaluation of research focused on underrepresented groups being key challenges. Intrinsic issues encompassed time management and grant writing, while personal struggles included balancing life and work and seeking social support.	EC, MC
Kippenbrock & Emory, 2021	Nursing	Quantitative research study	To determine NINR grant recipients' race/ethnicity, gender, and licensed nurse status.	In the survey, females, especially among licensed nurses, dominated as recipients. White people constituted the majority, with underrepresentation of Asian people and Black people. Notably, 47.6% of NINR grant recipients came from non-nursing backgrounds. The study revealed that nursing research funds often went to principal investigators (PIs) from other health disciplines, with a higher percentage of male PIs compared to licensed nurse grantees.	EC/MLC
Marriott et al., 2021	Biomedical science	Thematic analysis	Describes how enrichment was designed and implemented, including how it evolved over 30 months to better meet student needs.	Students appreciated the low-pressure, student-centered curriculum's goal to balance academic and research demands. The core themes of the enrichment program included community building, career path exploration, and professional identity development. The nonformal, interprofessional curricula allowed students to represent diverse biomedical identities and paths; informing institutional changes aimed at enhancing the success of diverse undergraduates in academia and research.	UG

(continued)

TABLE 4.2

Research Studies* (Continued)

Author(s), Year	Research Area	Type of Article	Study Aim(s)/Hypotheses	Outcomes	Level of Participants
Moore et al., 2017	Rehabilitation	Qualitative study	In what ways can federal research agencies, such as the NIDILRR; NIH; AHRQ; Office of Disability, Aging and Long-Term Care Policy; and others assist in building the pool of seasoned disability and health investigators from underrepresented groups?	Key informants stress the need for new career development pathways to address the shortage of experienced investigators from underrepresented groups. Engaging high school and college-level students is vital to raise awareness about research careers. Social justice concerns revolve around "discrimination," the persistent grant recycling to the same individuals, and a discouraging culture, necessitating an equity-first approach to combat bias. Targeted funding for investigators from underrepresented groups is crucial to expand their ranks, and mentorship programs play a pivotal role. Role models in research leadership are essential for investigators from underrepresented groups. Sponsorships at conferences targeting underrepresented ethnic groups can increase the pool of experienced researchers from underrepresented groups.	EC

Source	Field	Study type	Objective	Findings	
National Institutes of Health, 2022	Biomedical science	Quantitative research study	To show the latest funding rates and personal demographic data for principal investigators (PIs) for research program grant (RPG) applicants.	Between 2010 and 2021, R01 grant PIs were predominantly White (56%), followed by Asian (24%), unknown (12%), Hispanic (5%), and Black (3%). While Black and Hispanic applicants remained low, there was a notable increase in their numbers. Funding rates for Black PIs have increased, and Hispanic PIs have seen a smaller increase. White, Asian, and Hispanic PIs have risen but slightly decreased since 2020, nearing parity with Black PIs' increased rates.	EC/MLC
Rubio et al., 2019	Biomedical science	Qualitative focus groups research	Identify areas of training and support that would help junior investigators at institutions of higher education that serve underrepresented groups to develop and sustain research careers.	Four areas in which training and support were needed: training in the "informal curriculum" (skills not covered in traditional clinical research courses), protected time for research training, opportunities to create career-advancing work products, and networking opportunities. Identified themes informed the development of the LEADS (Leading Emerging and Diverse Scientists to Success) program.	EC
Shihabuddin et al., 2022	Pediatrics	Quantitative research study	Describe the characteristics of Clinical Research Coordinators in a large collaborative research network.	(26.4%) identified as UIM (Black, Hispanic, or Latino). Majority were White (65%), female (77%), 30 years and under (90%), 57% had a bachelor's degree. About 25% of respondents were from UIM, lower than the UIM population of the United States, but higher than the number of UIM in the U.S. health care workforce.	HS, UG, G

(continued)

TABLE 4.2

Research Studies* (Continued)

Author(s), Year	Research Area	Type of Article	Study Aim(s)/Hypotheses	Outcomes	Level of Participants
Sopher et al., 2015	HIV Research	Mixed methods program evaluation	Evaluation of the first 2 RAMP cohorts (2011–2013).	13 medical students completed RAMP; 62% were male, with 54% identifying as African American and 46% as Hispanic. The majority (54%) were in their first or second year of medical school. Projects were either short term (77%, lasting 8 to 16 weeks) or year-long (23%). Scholars reported increased knowledge of HIV research concepts and professional skills. Success factors included engaged mentors, comprehensive program administration, and sufficient funding for scholars' clinical site time and research expenses.	G
Thakar et al., 2023	Biomedical science	Pre-post-comparison quantitative	Examined associations of perseverance and consistency of interest with Clinical Research Appraisal Inventory (CRAI), science identity, effort–reward imbalance, and burnout, which may be related to career success.	The cohort comprises 80% females, 34% Hispanic/Latinx, and 33% non-Hispanic/Latinx Black individuals. It consists of 59% PhD researchers, 32% physician-scientists, and 8% with other higher degrees, with a median age of 37. Their median grit score is 3.8, signifying high perseverance. Physician-scientists, while similar in many aspects, have more years since their highest degree and lower grit scores. Greater perseverance and consistency of interest are linked to a stronger science identity, while lower consistency of interest relates to higher professional effort for fewer rewards. Both grit subscales associate with a robust science identity in UR post-doctoral fellows and early-career faculty.	PD/EC

Thoman et al., 2015	Biomedical science	Quantitative descriptive	Is there variability across students' perceptions of altruistic affordances for their research, predicting greater psychological involvement in their research laboratory and more interest in a scientific career?	Greater altruistic affordance predicted higher psychological involvement ($\beta = .37$; $p = .02$) and career interest ($\beta = .39$; $p = .006$) in students from underrepresented groups but not in White students. Students from under-represented groups perceiving high altruistic affordance were 3.32 times more likely to be highly involved in laboratory work and 2.55 times more likely to have strong career interest. This suggests that students from underrepresented groups who see their research as fulfilling altruistic goals are more engaged in research and more inclined to pursue careers in science.	UG
Thorpe et al., 2020	Biomedical science	Quantitative research study	NRMN STAR grant writing self-efficacy of trainees 12 months following completion.	Grantsmanship training—The NRMN STAR trainees improved grant writing self-efficacy from pre-assessment to the 12-month post-assessment. More than half the trainees were assistant professors (52%) and had none or less than 1 year of research experience beyond postdoctoral training (57%). However, 24% of the trainees reported no postdoctoral research training, and 29% were employed at minority serving institutions.	EC

(continued)

TABLE 4.2

Research Studies* (*Continued*)

Author(s), Year	Research Area	Type of Article	Study Aim(s)/Hypotheses	Outcomes	Level of Participants
Wiley et al., 2020	Biomedical science	Quantitative research study	Determine how representation from underrepresented groups changes over time. Identify characteristics associated with graduates from underrepresented groups that predict being successful.	Overall, 82.3% of respondents accepted academic positions. Hispanic respondents (89.2%) accepted at higher rates than all other racial groups ($p < .001$). Black doctoral recipients were marginally less likely to accept academic jobs. Graduates from underrepresented groups were more often single, with dependents and U.S. citizens. They also had more training in computer science or health compared to bioinformatics. Among academics from underrepresented groups, fewer graduated from private universities compared to public ones.	F
Williams et al., 2016	Biomedical science	Controlled study of program to increased diversity.	Hypotheses: The Academy group will have increased perceived achievability and desirability of an academic career.	No significant initial difference in perceived desirability of an academic career between men and women or between people from underrepresented groups and those not from underrepresented groups. Initially, female students and students from underrepresented groups did not differ from males and people not from underrepresented groups regarding academic career desirability. However, Academy students exhibited significantly improved perceptions about the attainability of an academic career.	G

Yoon et al., 2019	Behavioral science	Quantitative research study	To quantify how NIH-trained first authors have diversified across the past five decades.	A majority of T-32 training grants were centered on cardiovascular behavioral medicine, led by 70% males and 30% females, with just 7% being African American. Trends indicated a rise in Black male and White female leadership and a decrease in White male leadership. Among 4,302 publications, only 8% focused on race or ethnicity.	T32 investigators—EC
Zhou et al., 2021	Medicine	Mixed-methods program evaluation	Describe the initial outcomes from delivery of PASS programs to more students.	Participants were all from underrepresented groups. Six participants were returning students who had participated in the in-person PASS program the previous summer of 2019, while 9 students were first-time participants of the program. Respondents' self-reported competence in their ability to do research increased significantly after this summer of PASS.	UG

Note: NIH, National Institutes of Health; NINR, National Institute of Nursing Research; PI, principal investigator; UR, undergraduate; UIM, underrepresented in medicine; DEI, diversity, equity, and inclusion; CTSA, Clinical & Translational Science Awards (CTSA) program; BMS, biomedical science; NIDILRR, National Institute on Disability, Independent Living, and Rehabilitation Research; AHRQ, Agency for Healthcare Research and Quality.

*Note: In this table, the word "male" refers to a person assigned male at birth, and the word "female" refers to a person assigned female at birth.

TABLE 4.3

Patterns Identified in Review

Pattern	Advances	Gaps	Evidence for Practice	Research Recommendations
1. Majority of programs in literature are at the researcher level.	There were 26 programs that were described at the early-career researcher and graduate student level.	Limited evidence of LT effectiveness of graduate and earlier-stage programs.	Programs at the graduate student and early-career researcher levels demonstrate effective outcomes.	Approaches to increasing diversity at earlier student levels, such as high school and undergraduate levels, should be studied.
2. Some areas are well represented, while others are not.	Several medical specialties, especially HIV research programs, are represented. Institutions of higher education that serve underrepresented groups are a leader in this field.	Nursing, specialty medicine programs, SW, PH, and other. Interdisciplinary groups lack description of programs.	Extramural funding for programs with a plan for sustainability is important for program longevity.	Approaches to increasing diversity in nursing, social work, public health, and interdisciplinary biomedical research fields are needed.
3. Evaluation data of programs are often self-reported.	Measures of productivity are the most common objective measures.	More objective measures of program evaluation are needed.		Identify more objective measures in program evaluation.
4. Mentoring is a strong focus in all programs.	Mentoring as a tool is well documented as effective in supporting retention of diversity in biomedical researchers.		Mentoring is a hallmark of an effective program to increase diversity in biomedical research.	
5. Other areas of diversity	Most programs for diversity in biomedical research are focused on racial diversity.	Discussed very rarely— although more often in the past 5 years		More aspects of diversity should be addressed in both programs and research.

LT, long term; SW, social work; PH, public health.

for participation in research, and continuing into college where students can engage with researchers in health and biomedical fields to gain a deeper understanding of the wide range of career possibilities available to them. It is essential to recognize that conducting research in practice settings, such as nurses improving the quality of care or physical therapists exploring new modalities, does not necessitate functioning as a full-time researcher. Identifying ways for health care professionals in practice to collaborate with those possessing research expertise can broaden the scope of questions, studies, and conclusions that can be drawn from research endeavors. Moreover, community-based participatory research is highlighted as a promising approach in Chapter 3. This methodology involves engaging diverse perspectives within the research process to better address the needs of various populations. This approach can be a powerful tool for promoting inclusivity and equity in research initiatives.

Limitations

There were several limitations to this work. First, due to the large amount of literature, this study was limited to the past 10 years, which allowed the most current literature to be included. Although not limited by location, all articles in this review were conducted in the United States, so these results are not generalizable to other countries. The studies often relied on self-report, which is a limitation of the scholarship in this area. Finally, a single author abstracted and analyzed the data, so future reviews will need to confirm the reliability of the findings.

Exemplar Conclusion

Development of programs to diversify the biomedical research workforce are needed. Health equity is dependent on a diverse research workforce that can ask the questions, design and implement the studies, and interpret the results through an equity lens. A hallmark of programs to increase diversity is mentoring. In addition, most programs include mentored research experiences. Many programs also provided additional training, including grantsmanship, research skills, and peer support. Programs to increase diversity in the biomedical research workforce were most often conducted by institutions of higher education that serve underrepresented groups. The studies that examined the current state of diversity in the research workforce revealed continuing inequities for people of color and women. Overall, bias was found in NIH award scoring, although one study did not identify bias.

EXEMPLAR 2: RACISM IN NURSING: BIBLIOMETRIC ANALYSIS OF RACISM IN PUBLISHED NURSING SCIENTIFIC LITERATURE

Once research has been conducted to contribute to the knowledge about SSDH and strategies to address SSDH, barriers may arise during the dissemination of this research through publication. A study was conducted to identify biases in nursing publications. Racism is a pervasive problem that profoundly impacts the nursing profession. It manifests in various ways, including wage disparities, workplace harassment and bullying, limited opportunities for publishing in scholarly journals, and individuals being passed over for career advancement opportunities (ANA, 2021). The *Future of Nursing 2020–2030* report, released in 2021, envisions all nurses to be prepared "to meet the challenges associated with...structural racism" (p. 2, Box 5-1). The report further identified that the nursing profession has a history of racism and that nursing leaders must acknowledge historical racism and work to eliminate structural racism within the profession (p. 11). Racism not only affects care provided to historically underrepresented populations, including people of color who bear the burden of disproportionate illness rates, but also contributes to the lack of diversity in the nursing profession, which remains predominantly of European descent (Smiley et al., 2021).

Within the profession of nursing, a reluctance to come to terms with racism is posited to be due to three factors: 1) identity of Euro-American nurses as caring and, therefore, not seeing color of patient's skin, 2) a preference for homogeneity to promote efficiency, and 3) avoidance of conflict (Barbee, 1993). These factors, along with blatant racism at some places and points in history, have prevented those in the profession of nursing from confronting the racism within practice, education, and research.

Overview of Racism in U.S. Nursing History

Throughout its history, the nursing profession has grappled with the pervasive issue of racism. When nursing emerged in the late 19th century in the United States, racial discrimination was deeply entrenched in the profession. In northern states, nursing schools enforced racial quotas, and in the southern states, Black women were systematically denied admission to nursing schools (Rollins, 2022). In response to this discriminatory landscape, nurses of color advocated for change in the 1970s, leading to the formation of organizations such as the National Black Nurses Association (NBNA) and the National Association of Hispanic Nurses (NAHN) (Bennett et al., 2019). These associations aimed to address the specific needs and aspirations of nurses from diverse backgrounds, contributing to the advancement of the profession (Bennett et al., 2019).

Racism in nursing was not confined to a particular era or region. In 1879, Mary Eliza Mahoney became the first Black nurse to successfully complete a formal nursing program, but despite her groundbreaking achievement, she faced persistent discrimination and ultimately chose to leave the nursing profession (Davis, 1999; Oncology Nursing Society, 2021). In 1925, Ethel Johns, a nurse from Canada, extensively documented the prevailing racism across the United States (Davis, 1999; Oncology Nursing Society, 2021). Substantial progress was made following the desegregation of the military, including the Nurses Corps, in 1948. This milestone prompted nursing associations to revise bylaws and to eliminate membership exclusions based on race (Davis, 1999; Oncology Nursing Society, 2021).

The American Nurses Association (ANA) is actively involved in addressing racism issues and promoting diversity, equity, and inclusion within the nursing profession (ANA, 2022). The ANA recognizes the importance of acknowledging historical injustices and working toward a more equitable future. They have issued various statements, guidelines, and policies addressing these concerns. One such work is the ANA Racial Reckoning Statement, released on June 11, 2022, in which the ANA apologized for past actions contributing to systemic racism. The statement, which highlights specific instances of discriminatory practices leading to the exclusion of Black nurses, serves as a first step for the ANA to acknowledge its past actions and their negative impact on nurses of color (ANA, 2022).

In 2021, prominent nursing organizations established The National Commission to Address Racism in Nursing, led by the ANA, NBNA, NHNA, and the National Coalition of Ethnic Minority Nurse Associations (ANA, 2021). This Commission is undertaking an extensive investigation into the pervasive issue of racism within the nursing profession nationwide, with a specific focus on its impact on nurses, patients, communities, and health care systems (ANA, 2021). The Commission has published a series of reports on racism in nursing, covering topics such as the experiences of nurses of color throughout U.S. history; systemic racism in a contemporary society; and racism in policy, nursing education, practice, and research (ANA, 2022; National Commission to Address Racism in Nursing, 2021). These reports collectively aim to inspire and motivate all nurses to actively address both individual and systemic forms of racism.

Although the Commission acknowledges systemic racism in all nursing spaces, including education, practice, and policy, the discussion here will focus on the pervasive nature of racism in publishing. Recent calls for changes in publishing practices in the medical field have been highlighted in articles by Boyd et al. (2020); Krieger et al. (2021); Merchant et al. (2021); Salazar et al. (2021); Liu et al. (2023). Now, it is time for the nursing publishing industry to do the same. The objective of this study is to gain a deeper understanding of the scope and trends in the nursing literature related to racism.

Methods

Three different phases of bibliometric analysis were chosen to first identify trends in the broader health care literature on the topic of racism using PubMed, then to conduct a manual search of the top 20 nursing journals by impact factor to identify how often the most impactful journals published articles with the word "racism" as a keyword or within the title, and finally to conduct an analysis using Dimensions AI, a more complete citation database than PubMed, to visualize the data and to perform more sophisticated analyses.

Phases 1 and 2

This study employed a bibliometric analysis approach with multiple phases to identify the trends in health care, and then nursing literature, on the topic of racism. Bibliometric analysis was chosen because the topic of study was trends in the literature. First, PubMed was searched for the term "racism" for the 10-year period between 2013 and 2022 to identify general trends in health care literature. PubMed is an open-source database that provides free access to articles that describe federally funded research (National Library of Medicine, 2023).

To focus on the most impactful nursing literature, the second phase in our analysis consisted of conducting a manual search of the past 10 years of issues of the top 20 nursing journals by impact factor (Clarivate, 2023). *Impact factor* is a measure of how often articles within a journal are cited by other authors; although it is controversial due to skewed distributions of citation counts, it does provide a journal measure of the collective importance of the articles included in a journal. The manual search was conducted by three researchers for the word "racism" in the article title or as a keyword in each journal between January 2013 and December 2022 to identify the number of articles on racism published per year.

Phase 3

The third phase of the study employed methods for bibliometric analysis suggested by Zupic and Cater (2015). In step 1 of the workflow, a bibliometric analysis approach, including data visualization, was used to identify the scope of scholarly literature with the keyword "racism" over a 10-year period. That time period was chosen because discussion of racism in health care is a relatively recent phenomenon. Bibliometrics allows for questions that probe the intellectual structure or knowledge base, and the conceptual structure, or mapping of a scientific community around a specific topic (Aria & Cuccurullo, 2017).

In step 2 of the workflow for the analysis, bibliometric data is compiled. Dimensions AI (Digital Science, 2018), a bibliographic research database with over 137 million publications, was used to compile relevant citations. To elicit the maximum number of articles, the keyword "racism" was searched between 2013 and 2022. The documents were then limited to those in the "nursing" category. The 500 most relevant articles were selected because the Dimensions AI free access only allowed 500 sources to be downloaded. The raw files were uploaded into the biblioshiny app of the R bibliometrix program (Aria & Cuccurullo, 2017). Data were then cleaned, and missing data were identified.

Bibliometric data analysis, step 3, was conducted using bibliometrix (Aria & Cuccurullo, 2017), an R-tool, and the biblioshiny Web-based application. Descriptive analyses were conducted including number of publications per year, average citations per year, number of authors, and location and affiliation of authors. Data visualization, step 4, employed the use of biblioshiny, an app within bibliometrix. Scientific production by country, affiliation, and author production over time were all visualized to make sense of the data. Further conceptual analysis of the knowledge of racism in nursing publications was visualized using a factorial analysis multiple correspondence analysis approach and co-word analysis (Aria & Cuccurullo, 2017). Review by an Institutional Review Board was not sought because the study included published literature only and human participants were not included.

Data Synthesis

Table 4.4 summarizes the dataset information. The Dimension AI database produced a total of 503 articles in 161 distinct sources with the topic "racism" within the nursing category (of which the 500 most relevant articles were analyzed). The mean yearly production over the 10-year period was 50 (SD = 41.95; range: 16–64). Of these, there was little variation in the number of articles on the topic of racism between 2013 and 2018 (m = 22.33; SD = 3.08; range: 19–27), with a slight skew to the right (skewness = .70). In 2019, there was an almost doubling of the total number of publications from

TABLE 4.4

Data Synthesis and Summary of the Dataset

Description	Results
Sources (journals, books, etc.)	161
Time period	2013–2022
Documents	500
Annual growth rate %	29.51
Document average age	2.98
Average citations per document	9.42
Author's keywords	635
Authors ➤ Authors ➤ Authors of single-authored documents	 1,821 81
Authors Collaboration ➤ Single-authored documents ➤ Coauthors per document ➤ International coauthorships %	 89 4.42 5.8

the previous year, then in 2020 the number doubled again and continued to increase in 2021, leveling off in 2022 (see Figure 4.2). This trend can be seen in the average age of documents in the data, which is 2.98 years. The number of articles in each journal ranged from 1 to 34. *Nursing Inquiry* had the greatest number of articles per source (*n* = 34), followed by *Advances in Nursing Science* (*n* = 25), *Creative Nursing and Journal*

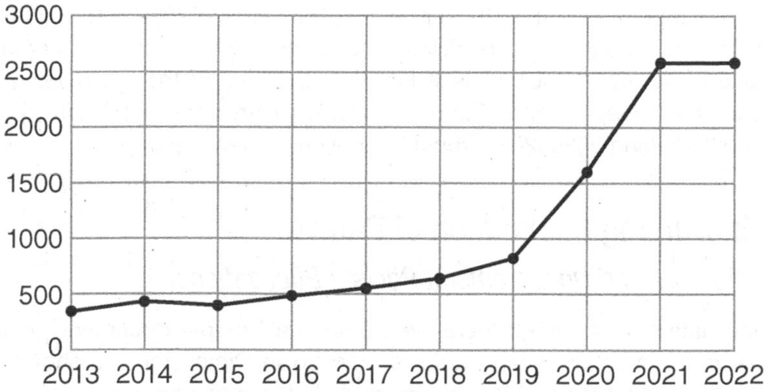

FIGURE 4.2 PubMed query "racism" between 2013 and 2022 (conducted June 16, 2023); publications per year with key word "racism."

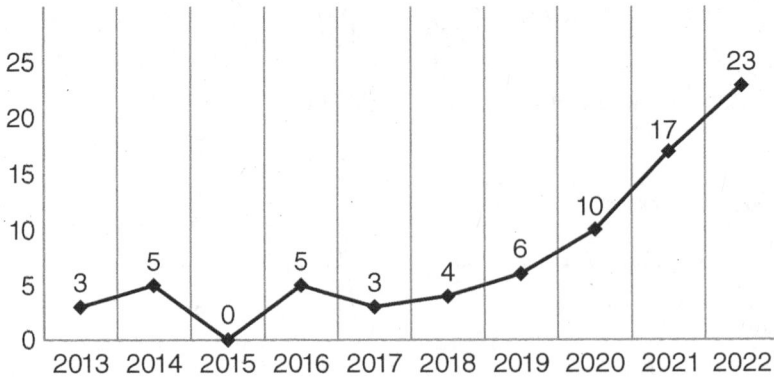

FIGURE 4.3 Top 20 nursing journals by impact factor with "racism" as a keyword or in the title by year.

of *Professional Nursing* ($n = 19$ each), and *Public Health Nursing* ($n = 18$). Most journals published only one article ($n = 94$) during the study period. The cited references, language, and number of cited references were not available from the dataset, so co-citation analysis was unable to be conducted. Data cleaning of author and affiliation names was conducted manually.

Results and Discussion

Growth of "Racism" as a Keyword

The results of the first phase of the analysis can be seen in Figure 4.2. The total number of articles with the topic "racism" in this 10-year period was 10,478. There was a sharp increase in articles indexed in PubMed with the term "racism" beginning in 2019 continuing through 2021 but leveling off in 2022. In Figure 4.3 the second-phase results, a similar pattern occurred but delayed by 1 year in the most cited nursing literature. As can be seen in Table 4.5, half of the journals either published only one article or no articles on this topic during the 10-year period. The years 2020, 2021, and 2022 were separated out because these years saw a substantial increase in the number of articles with the title or keyword "racism" (see Figure 4.3). Three of the top nursing journals (*Nurse Education Today*, *Nursing Outlook*, and *BMC Nursing*) saw an increase of three or more articles during 2020–2022 from the previous seven years.

Trends in Nursing Publication of Racism

Relevant Authors and Documents of Racism Publications

The citation data demonstrated there were 9.42 citations per document, on average. The annual production of nursing articles indexed in Dimensions AI shows a sharp increase between 2019 and 2021 (see Figure 4.4). The mean total number of citations per article has decreased over the past 10 years (see Table 4.6), although the mean number of total citations per year has remained relatively stable ($m = 2.52$; SD = .94). Six

TABLE 4.5

Journal Articles With "Racism" as a Keyword or in Title in Top 20 Nursing Journals

Journal Title (Impact Factor)	2013–2019	2020–2022
International Journal of Nursing Studies (6.6)	1	I
International Journal of Mental Health Nursing (5.1)	5	I.
Journal of Nursing Management (4.7)	0	I
Journal of Clinical Nursing (4.4)	5	5
Worldviews on Evidence-Based Nursing (4.3)	0	0
Intensive and Critical Care Nursing (4.2)	0	0
Journal of Nursing Scholarship (3.9)	2	2
Nurse Education Today (3.9)	3	12
European Journal of Cardiovascular Nursing (3.6)	0	0
Seminars in Oncology Nursing (3.5)	0	0
Nurse Education in Practice (3.4)	I	3
International Nursing Review (3.4)	0	1
Journal of Tissue Viability (3.4)	0	1
Women and Birth (3.3)	1	0
Nursing Ethics (3.3)	1	0
Nursing Outlook (3.3)	1	14
Australian Critical Care (3.3)	0	0
BMC Nursing (3.2)	0	3
Birth—Issues in Perinatal Care (3.1)	0	2
Journal of Advanced Nursing (3.1)	6	5

articles are cited between 12 and 7.5 times per year (see Table 4.7) and written by three authors. The range of total citations for these three articles is between 30 and 61. The total number of citations from all articles in the data set for Iheduru-Anderson is 157, followed by West with 120, and Waite with 109. These are arguably the most influential articles and authors on this topic in nursing.

There were 1,821 authors of the 500 documents, and 81 of these were authors of single-authored documents. The majority of documents were coauthored with an average of 4.42 coauthors per document. The most prolific authors were K. Iheduru-Anderson ($n = 10$) between 2018 and 2022, followed by R. West ($n = 8$), and K. Jeffries ($n = 8$), and R. Waite ($n = 6$). Iheduru-Anderson, Waite, and West are also the most cited authors total and per year in this dataset.

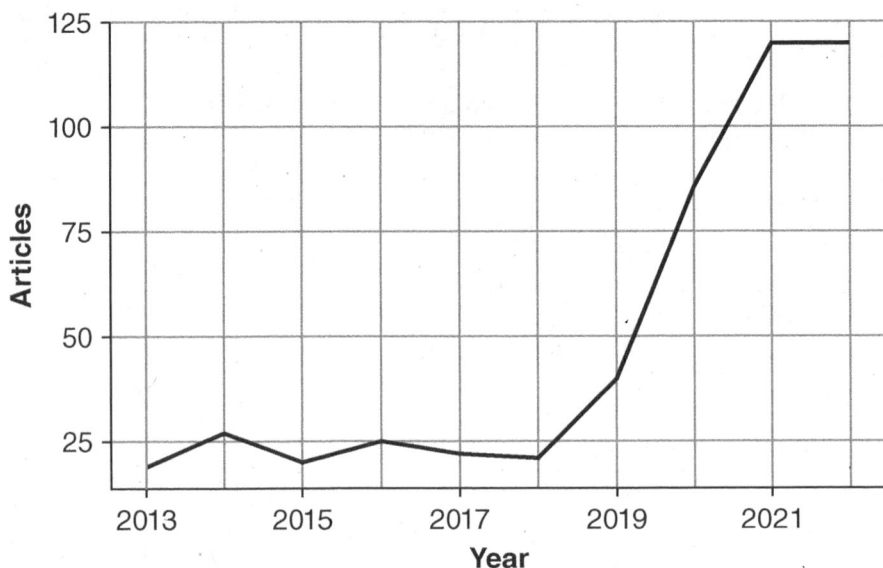

FIGURE 4.4 Annual scientific production indexed in Dimensions AI. (Created using *Bibliometrix/ Biblioshiny* software in R studio.)

	TABLE 4.6			
Mean Citations Per Article and Per Year				
Year	Mean Citations Per Article	Number	Mean Citations Per Year	Citable Years
2013	27.94	16	2.54	11
2014	14.65	17	1.47	10
2015	25.91	11	2.88	9
2016	21.1	20	2.64	8
2017	33.79	19	4.83	7
2018	17.17	18	2.86	6
2019	12.6	25	2.52	5
2020	10.75	60	2.69	4
2021	7.04	150	2.35	3
2022	2.09	164	1.04	2

TABLE 4.7

Most Cited Nursing Articles on Key Word "Racism"

Author	Year	Title	Journal	Total Citations	Citations Per Year
Waite, R.	2017	Nursing colonialism in America: implications for nursing leadership	*Journal of Professional Nursing*	61	8.71
West, R.	2020	A unified call to action from Australian nursing and midwifery leaders: ensuring that black lives matter	*Contemporary Nurse*	48	12
Waite, R.	2020	Achieving health equity through eradicating structural racism in the United States: a call to action for nursing leadership	*Journal of Nursing Scholarship*	33	8.25
Iheduru-Anderson, K.	2020	Discourse on race and racism in nursing: an integrative review of literature	*Public Health Nursing*	32	8
Iheduru-Anderson, K.	2020	The White/Black hierarchy institutionalizes White supremacy in nursing and nursing leadership in the United States	*Journal of Professional Nursing*	30	7.5
Iheduru-Anderson, K.	2020	Barriers to career advancement in the nursing profession: perceptions of Black nurses in the United States	*Nursing Forum*	30	7.5
Iheduru-Anderson, K.	2021	Rejecting the myth of equal opportunity: an agenda to eliminate racism in nursing education in the United States	*BMC Nursing*	18	6

Scientific Publication by Region and Affiliation

International coauthorships were rare with just 5.8% of documents. Figure 4.5 shows the country collaboration, and the darkness of gray denotes the number of authors from that country, with dark gray corresponding with the highest number. The United States had the most publications followed by Canada and Australia. There are 587 distinct affiliations within the database. Figure 4.6 displays the 20 affiliations that were most common. Affiliations included colleges and universities, health services, Aboriginal/First Nations health organizations, national centers, professional organizations,

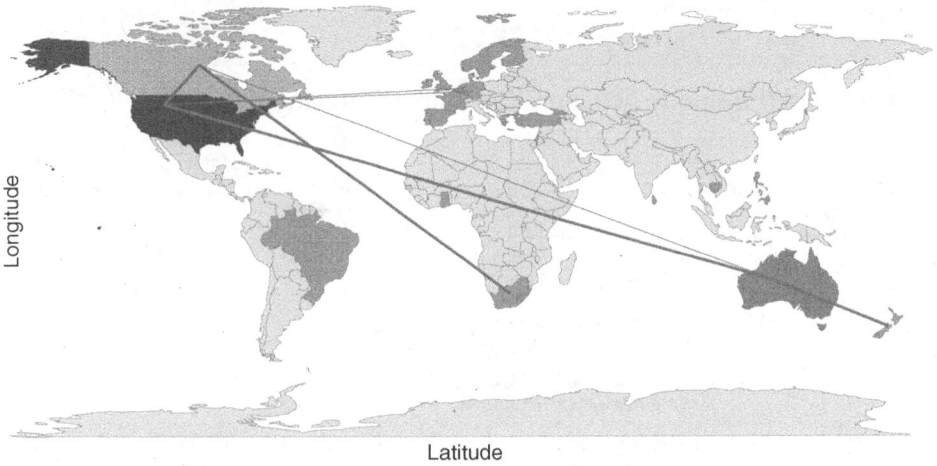

FIGURE 4.5 Country collaboration map. (Created using *Bibliometrix/Biblioshiny* software in R studio.)

institutes, public health departments, hospitals, managed care organizations, and individual businesses.

Keyword Analysis, Co-Occurrence Network, and Trend Topics

Scholars use keywords to quickly find relevant sources when conducting research (Corrin et al., 2022). An analysis of keywords can identify the trending topics and areas of focus (Corrin et al., 2022). The word cloud in Figure 4.7 visualizes the most commonly used keywords.

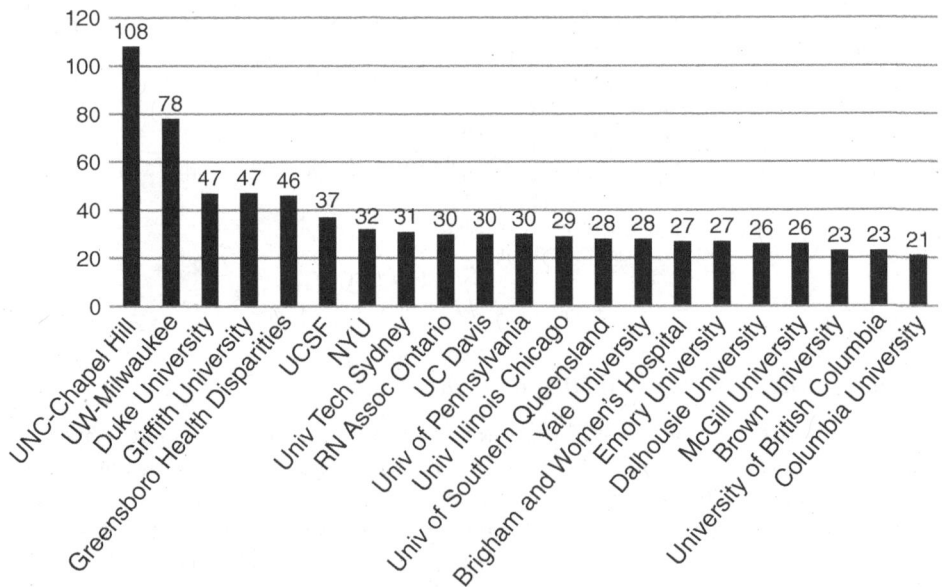

FIGURE 4.6 Number of articles by author affiliation.

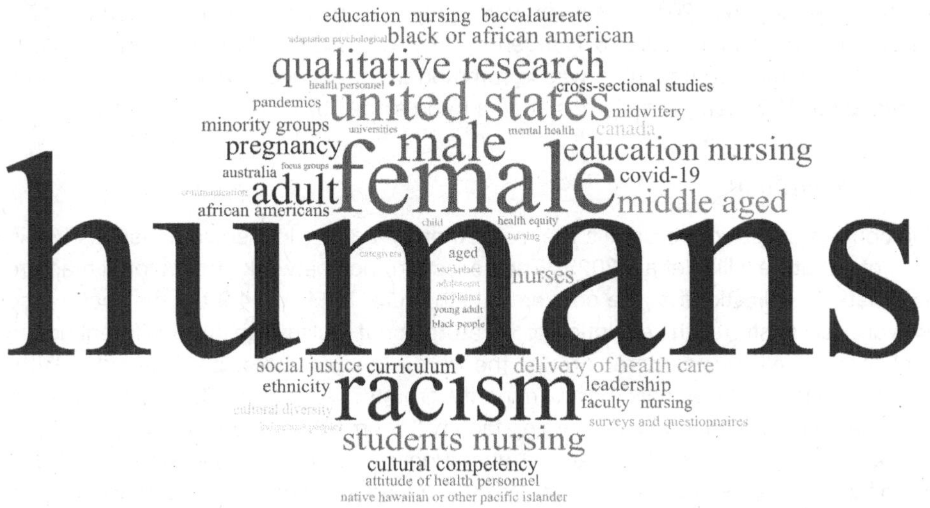

FIGURE 4.7 Word cloud. Note: In this figure, the word "male" refers to a person assigned male at birth, and the word "female" refers to a person assigned female at birth. (Created using *Bibliometrix/Biblioshiny* software in R studio.)

The analysis of trending topics is based upon commonly used keywords and demonstrates keyword use over time (see Figure 4.8). Within the analysis, the word minimum frequency was set at 5, with 5 words per year. Within this dataset, it is not until 2021 that the keyword "racism" is used an appreciable amount with a frequency of 200 that year,

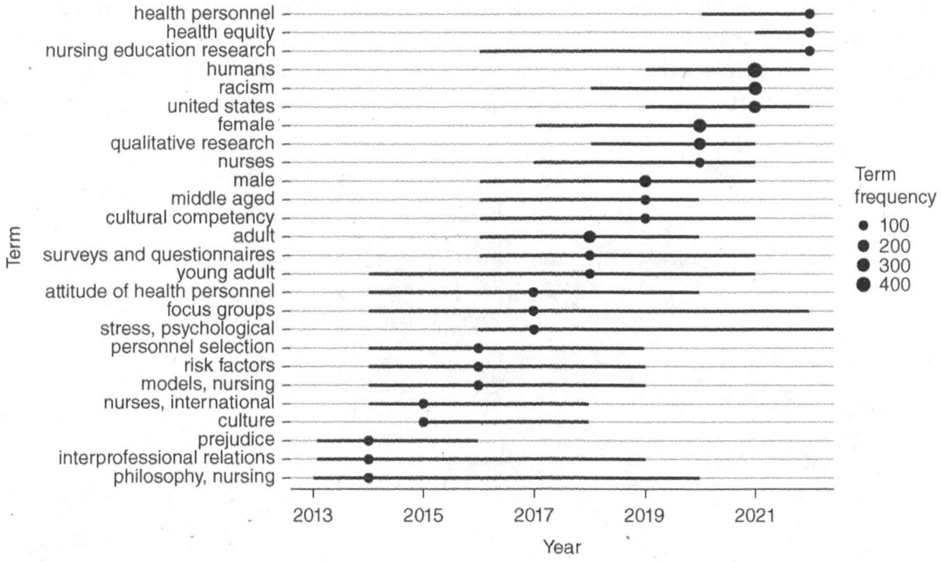

FIGURE 4.8 Trend topics within dataset. Note: In this figure, the word "male" refers to a person assigned male at birth, and the word "female" refers to a person assigned female at birth. (Created using *Bibliometrix/Biblioshiny* software in R studio.)

although use began in 2018. A similar word, prejudice, which connotes an individually-mediated form of bias (Salter & Haugen, 2017), was used more often between 2013 and 2016. Cultural competence was a common trend between 2016 and 2021 with a frequency of 100. Health equity has been a trend since 2021.

Data Visualization

The conceptual structure details the major themes and their associated issues within a set of literature (Ullah et al., 2023). The co-occurrence network and factorial map are both data visualizations of the conceptual structure. In Figure 4.9 the co-occurrence network demonstrates the evolution of literature about racism into three different nodes or clusters. The first is centered around the words "humans," "racism," "female," "attitude of health professionals," and "minority groups." At lower left, the terms "baccalaureate nursing education," "nursing faculty," "curriculum," "cultural competency," "social justice," "Native Hawaiian or other Pacific Islander," "indigenous peoples," "pregnancy," "midwifery," and "Australia," form a node. Another much smaller one (at lower right) is "COVID-19," "pandemics," "nursing," "leadership," and "health equity." The factorial map (Figure 4.10) provides a broad perspective on the topics associated with racism. Within the factorial map, the keywords are analyzed by multiple corresponding analysis (MCA) and how close keywords appear to one another indicates a shared meaning (Ullah et al., 2023). The key words "Covid-19," "pandemics," "health equity," and "delivery of health care" are close in proximity, indicating a large proportion of articles sharing these key words. Another cluster of key words is "racism," "health," "personal," "communication," "black people," "minority groups," and "health care disparities." "Nursing research," "nursing," and "leadership" are relatively close together. Although some terms are spaced far apart, within the concept of racism there are not separate topics that stand out. It is notable that words related to racism and interpersonal relationships such as "attitudes of health care professionals," "personal," "health personnel," and "health care delivery" are found in the co-occurrence

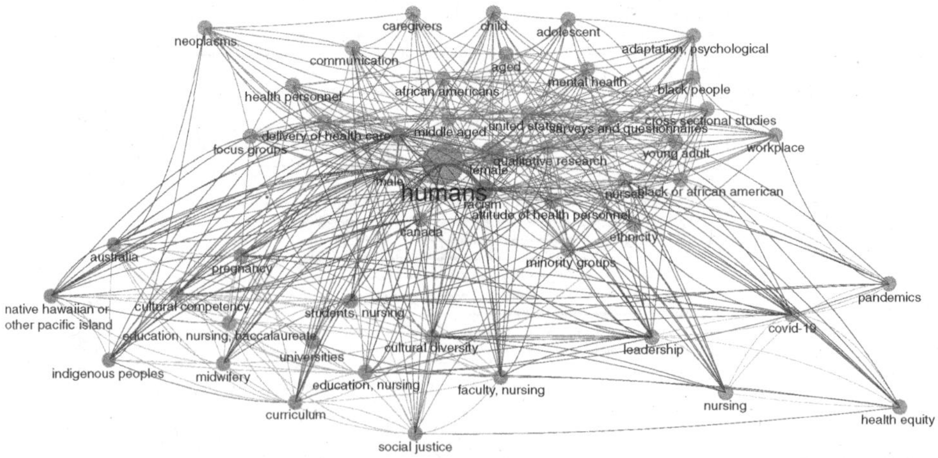

FIGURE 4.9 Co-occurrence network. Note: In this figure, the word "male" refers to a person assigned male at birth, and the word "female" refers to a person assigned female at birth. (Created using *Bibliometrix/Biblioshiny* software in R studio.)

Conceptual Structure Map - method: MCA

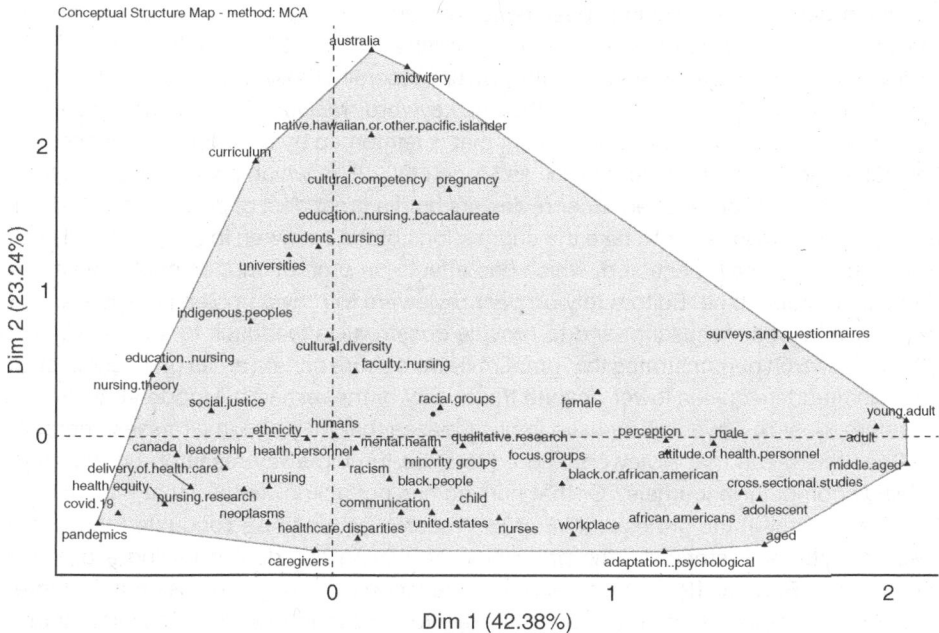

FIGURE 4.10 Factorial map. Note: In this figure, the word "male" refers to a person assigned male at birth, and the word "female" refers to a person assigned female at birth. (Created using *Bibliometrix/ Biblioshiny* software in R studio.)

network and the factorial map, but words that speak to institutionally mediated racism and social determinants of health are not found.

Limitations

Several limitations were present within this study. First, cited references in the documents were not available because the authors used a free, nonsubscription access dataset. This meant that co-citation analysis could not be conducted. The free, nonsubscription access also limited the dataset to only 500 documents with data that could be downloaded for use with the data visualization software. Fortunately for the study, this left out only three documents. Use of Web of Science or Scopus databases would have likely produced more complete data but was not available to the author conducting the bibliographic analysis with data visualization. The current study provides a baseline understanding of the scope of nursing scholarly literature about racism.

Exemplar Conclusion

Although there has been a dramatic increase in the number of articles focused on racism, nursing has been slower to follow this trend. The nursing journals that are cited most by impact factor are not publishing articles on racism as a general rule, with a few standouts. Racism is a powerful force and has led to health inequities through structural and social determinants of health (NASEM, 2021).

Within scholarly publishing, peer reviewers are important gatekeepers to assure the integrity and quality of science that is published (Chinn, 2020). Unfortunately, peer reviewers are reflective of people with power, generally those with greater degree of education, within the group. The fact that the keyword "racism" was not used until 2018 may be due to bias in peer review, a point that is reinforced by anecdotal experiences of several authors of this article, as well as Moceri (2022), in which reviewers objected to the word "racism" being used. Peer reviewers hold a great deal of power, and although an author can choose not to take the suggestions of the reviewer, in so doing, they risk their manuscript being rejected, which has effects on promotion, personal motivation, and considerable time. Editors rely on peer reviewers to provide objective assessment of the quality of a manuscript and to provide constructive feedback to authors (Chinn, 2020). Research demonstrates that grant reviewers score certain areas of research such as racism and inequities lower despite the quality of the research (Hoppe et al., 2019); therefore, peer reviewers likely have implicit biases that may alter their assessment.

Does this mean that reviewers and editors are turning away research on this topic in highly competitive journals? Or that nursing has not acknowledged that racism is an important factor in the profession? Further research needs to be conducted to answer these questions. Historically, the profession of nursing has denied having a problem with racism (Barbee, 1993) because of our identity as a caring profession and, therefore, the assumption that nurses are not likely to behave in this way. Research shows that racism—interpersonal, implicit bias, and structural—does play a significant role in health inequities and that the nursing profession is part of the cause of health inequities (National Commission to Address Racism in Nursing, 2021). It is critical to examine the topic of racism in health care to achieve health equity. Therefore, the stall in the upward trajectory of publishing on this topic in health care between 2021 and 2022 is concerning because it could signal a decrease in the perceived importance of this topic to health care and nursing literature. On the other hand, there was not a flattening of the rise in publications in the nursing literature between 2021 and 2022, which is a hopeful sign. The profession of nursing is taking steps to face racism through ANA's Racial Reckoning Statement and the National Commission to Address Racism in Nursing, but there is still significant room for growth in the research and publishing sectors. Racism is the root of structural barriers that lead to health inequities. Without facing racism's roots in all areas of nursing, we cannot achieve health equity, because if our roots are diseased, the plant cannot thrive.

CONCLUSION AND CALL TO ACTION

In this chapter, two exemplars of research and dissemination issues related to SSDH were provided. Through a comprehensive scoping review of diversity in the biomedical research workforce and initiatives to enhance diversity, mentoring emerged as a cornerstone of successful programs to diversify this workforce. Additionally, mentored research experiences and supplementary training in grant management, research skills, and peer review were recognized as essential. Diversifying the biomedical research workforce produces a variety of perspectives and approaches to scientific inquiry. This diversity leads to innovative solutions to health equity issues, as different perspectives can identify research questions, propose scientific methods, and interpret findings in unique ways.

The second exemplar focuses on the historical context of racism in nursing and the challenges of addressing it in scholarly literature. While explicit exclusion based on race in nursing education and professional associations has diminished over time, structural barriers persist in various aspects of nursing, including education, practice, and policy. Until recently, there has been a reluctance to publish manuscripts addressing racism in nursing, leading to a limited body of literature on the topic. This reluctance may be attributed to implicit biases among reviewers and editors. However, there are signs of progress, such as initiatives by organizations like the International Academy of Nurse Editors to address biases in peer review and editing (American Nurses Association, 2024). This supports an urgent need to expand nursing scholarship on the effects of racism on practice, policy, and education. By fostering a deeper understanding of these issues, nursing can take meaningful actions to combat racism as a determinant of health.

These exemplars emphasize the importance of diversity and equity in research and practice within the biomedical and nursing fields. They highlight the need for ongoing efforts to address structural barriers, promote inclusivity, and expand scholarly dialogue on critical issues such as racism.

In response to the pressing need for action within the nursing profession, nurses must unite to promote diversity, equity, and inclusion in all nursing spaces. Recognizing the critical importance of these values, nurses should commit to fostering a nursing community that embraces individuals from all backgrounds and identities. To achieve this, nurses must champion mentorship programs that support aspiring nursing professionals from diverse backgrounds, recognizing mentoring as a cornerstone of effective programs to diversify the workforce. Furthermore, nurses should pledge to amplify the voices of their colleagues of color who have been historically underrepresented or silenced, particularly regarding issues of racism in nursing. By creating spaces for open dialogue and supporting initiatives that encourage nurses to share their experiences and insights, nurses are uniquely positioned to drive meaningful change. Nurses should also support initiatives that challenge implicit biases within nursing scholarship and publishing. Moreover, nurses must recognize the urgent need to expand nursing scholarship on the effects of racism on practice, policy, and education. By generating more evidence and discourse on this critical issue, nurses can build a stronger foundation for nursing actions to eliminate racism as a determinant of health. Additionally, nurses are responsible for advocating for structural changes within nursing education, practice, and policy to dismantle barriers that perpetuate inequities. Through their commitment to continuous learning and improvement, nurses will drive positive change within the profession and the broader health care system, ensuring that every nurse can thrive and contribute to improving the health and well-being of all individuals and communities.

Challenging Thoughts to Consider

1. What examples can you detail that frame the importance of research in the dissemination and shifting public thinking related to health, equity, and racism?

2. What are the indicators or "hallmarks" of programs to increase diversity in the educational programs, research, and practice environments?

3. What are outcomes to be reached that foster the ongoing profession of nursing to remain leaders in the advocacy and provision of equitable health care to all persons and populations?

References

Abebe, K. Z., Morone, N. E., Mayowski, C. A., Rubio, D. M., & Kapoor, W. K. (2019). Sowing the "CEED"s of a more diverse biomedical workforce: The Career Education and Enhancement for Health Care Research Diversity (CEED) program at the University of Pittsburgh. *Journal of Clinical and Translational Science*, *3*(1), 21—26. https://doi.org/10.1017/cts.2019.364

Amaechi, O., Foster, K. E., Tumin, D., & Campbell, K. M. (2021). Addressing the gate blocking of minority faculty. *Journal of the National Medical Association*, *113*(5), 517–521. https://doi.org/10.1016/j.jnma.2021.04.002

American Nurses Association. (2021, April 6). *National Commission to Address Racism in Nursing* [Professional Organization]. ANA. https://www.nursingworld.org/practice-policy/workforce/racism-in-nursing/national-commission-to-address-racism-in-nursing/

American Nurses Association. (2022, July 11). *Our Racial Reckoning Statement*. American Nurses Association. https://www.nursingworld.org/practice-policy/workforce/racism-in-nursing/RacialReckoningStatement/

American Nurses Association. (2024, January 18). *The National Commission to Address Racism in Nursing awards $200,000 to efforts committed to dismantling racism in nursing in 2024*. https://www.nursingworld.org/news/news-releases/2024/commission-rfp-winners/

Andriole, D. A., & Jeffe, D. B. (2016). Predictors of full-time faculty appointment among MD-PhD program graduates: A national cohort study. *Medical Education Online*, *21*, 30941. https://doi.org/10.3402/meo.v21.30941

Andriole, D. A., Yan, Y., & Jeffe, D. B. (2017). Mediators of racial/ethnic disparities in mentored K award receipt among U.S. medical school graduates. *Academic Medicine*, *92*(10), 1440–1448. https://doi.org/10.1097/ACM.0000000000001871

Aria, M., & Cuccurullo, C. (2017). bibliometrix: An R-tool for comprehensive science mapping analysis. *Journal of Informetrics*, *11*(4), 959–975. https://doi.org/10.1016/j.joi.2017.08.007

Arksey, H., & O'Malley, L. (2005). Scoping studies: Towards a methodological framework. *International Journal of Social Research Methodology*, *8*(1), 19–32. https://doi.org/10.1080/1364557032000119616

Awad, C. S., Deng, Y., Kwagyan, J., Roche-Lima, A., Tchounwou, P. B., Wang, Q., & Idris, M. Y. (2022). Summary of year-one effort of the RCMI Consortium to enhance research capacity and diversity with data science. *International Journal of Environmental Research and Public Health*, *20*(1), 279. https://doi.org/10.3390/ijerph20010279

Barbee, E. L. (1993). Racism in U.S. nursing. *Medical Anthropology Quarterly*, *7*(4), 346–362.

Bennett, C., Hamilton, E. K., & Rochani, H. (2019). Exploring racism in nursing: Teaching nursing students about racial inequality using the historical lens. *OJIN The Online Journal of Issues in Nursing*, *24*(2). https://doi.org/10.3912/OJIN.Vol24No02PPT20

Board on Population Health and Public Health Practice, Health and Medicine Division, & National Academies of Sciences, Engineering, and Medicine. (2016). *Framing the dialogue on race and ethnicity to advance health equity: Proceedings of a workshop*, (D.Thompson, Ed.). National Academies Press. https://www.nap.edu/catalog/23576

Boyd, R. W., Lindo, E. G., Weeks, L. D., & McLemore, M. R. (2020). On racism: A new standard for publishing on racial health inequities. *Health Affairs Forefront*. https://doi.org/10.1377/forefront.20200630.939347

Boyington, J. E. A., Maihle, N. J., Rice, T. K., Gonzalez, J. E., Hess, C. A., Makala, L. H., Jeffe, D. B., Ogedegbe, G., Rao, D. C., Dávila-Román, V. G., Pace, B. S., Jean-Louis, G., & Boutjdir, M. (2016). A perspective on promoting diversity in the biomedical research workforce: The National Heart, Lung, and Blood Institute's PRIDE program. *Ethnicity & Disease*, *26*(3), 379. https://doi.org/10.18865/ed.26.3.379

Bradbury-Jones, C., Aveyard, H., Herber, O. R., Isham, L., Taylor, J., & O'Malley, L.

(2022). Scoping reviews: The PAGER framework for improving the quality of reporting. *International Journal of Social Research Methodology, 25*(4), 457–470. https://doi.org/10.1080/13645579.2021.1899596

Brandon, D. H., Collins-McNeil, J., Onsomu, E. O., & Powell, D. L. (2014). Winston-Salem State University and Duke University's Bridge to the Doctorate Program. *North Carolina Medical Journal, 75*(1), 68–70. https://doi.org/10.18043/ncm.75.1.68

Brenner, M. J., Nelson, R. F., Valdez, T. A., Moody-Antonio, S. A., Nathan, C.-A. O., St John, M. A., & Francis, H. W. (2022). Centralized otolaryngology research efforts: Stepping-stones to innovation and equity in otolaryngology-head and neck surgery. *Otolaryngology—Head and Neck Surgery, 166*(6), 1192–1195. https://doi.org/10.1177/01945998211065465

Butler, J., 3rd, Fryer, C. S., Ward, E., Westaby, K., Adams, A., Esmond, S. L., Garza, M. A., Hogle, J. A., Scholl, L. M., Quinn, S. C., Thomas, S. B., & Sorkness, C. A. (2017). The Health Equity Leadership Institute (HELI): Developing workforce capacity for health disparities research. *Journal of Clinical and Translational Science, 1*(3), 153–159. https://doi.org/10.1017/cts.2017.6

Canner, J. E., McEligot, A. J., Pérez, M.-E., Qian, L., & Zhang, X. (2017). Enhancing diversity in biomedical data science. *Ethnicity & Disease, 27*(2), 107–116. https://doi.org/10.18865/ed.27.2.107

Chinn, P. L. (2020). Becoming a peer reviewer. *Nurse Author & Editor, 30*(3), 2–3. https://doi.org/10.1111/nae2.1

Clarivate. (2023). 2022 Journal Impact Factor. *Journal Citation Reports*. https://jcr.clarivate.com/jcr/home

Coghlan, D., & Brydon-Miller, M. (Eds.). (2014). *The SAGE encyclopedia of action research*. Sage Publications Limited.

Corrin, L., Thompson, K., Hwang, G.-J., & Lodge, J. M. (2022). The importance of choosing the right keywords for educational technology publications. *Australasian Journal of Educational Technology, 38*(2), 1–8. https://doi.org/10.14742/ajet.8087

Crockett, E. T. (2014). A research education program model to prepare a highly qualified workforce in biomedical and health-related research and increase diversity. *BMC Medical Education, 14*, 202. https://doi.org/10.1186/1472-6920-14-202

Croff, R., Tang, W., Friedman, D. B., Balbim, G. M., & Belza, B. (2022). Training the next generation of aging and cognitive health researchers. *Gerontology & Geriatrics Education, 43*(2), 185–201. https://doi.org/10.1080/02701960.2020.1824912

Crump, C., Ned, J., & Winkleby, M. A. (2015). The Stanford Medical Youth Science Program: Educational and science-related outcomes. *Advances in Health Sciences Education, 20*(2), 457–466. https://doi.org/10.1007/s10459-014-9540-6

Davis, A. T. (1999). *Early black American leaders in nursing: Architects for integration and equality*. Jones & Bartlett Publishers.

Digital Science. (2018). *Dimensions* [Computer software]. https://app.dimensions.ai

Doyle, J. M., Morone, N. E., Proulx, C. N., Althouse, A. D., Rubio, D. M., Thakar, M. S., Murrell, A. J., & White, G. E. (2021). The impact of the COVID-19 pandemic on underrepresented early-career PhD and physician scientists. *Journal of Clinical and Translational Science, 5*(1), e174. https://doi.org/10.1017/cts.2021.851

Duffus, W. A., Trawick, C., Moonesinghe, R., Tola, J., Truman, B. I., & Dean, H. D. (2014). Training racial and ethnic minority students for careers in public health sciences. *American Journal of Preventive Medicine, 47*(5), S368–S375. https://doi.org/10.1016/j.amepre.2014.07.028

Duncan, G. A., Lockett, A., Villegas, L. R., Almodovar, S., Gomez, J. L., Flores, S. C., Wilkes, D. S., & Tigno, X. T. (2016). National Heart, Lung, and Blood Institute Workshop Summary: Enhancing opportunities for training and retention of a diverse biomedical workforce. *Annals of the American Thoracic Society, 13*(4), 562–567. https://doi.org/10.1513/AnnalsATS.201509-624OT

Duong, J., McIntosh, S., Attia, J., Michener, J. L., Cottler, L. B., & Aguilar-Gaxiola, S. A. (2023). Attitudes towards diversity, equity, and inclusion across the CTSA Programs: Strong but not uniform support and commitment. *Journal of Clinical and Translational Science, 7*(1), e66. https://doi.org/10.1017/cts.2022.525

Erosheva, E. A., Grant, S., Chen, M.-C., Lindner, M. D., Nakamura, R. K., & Lee, C. J. (2020). NIH peer review: Criterion scores completely account for racial disparities in overall impact scores. *Science Advances, 6*(23), eaaz4868. https://doi.org/10.1126/sciadv.aaz4868

Estape, E. S., Quarshie, A., Segarra, B., San Martin, M., Ríos, R., Martínez, K., Ali, J., Nwagwu, U., Ofili, E., & Pemu, P. (2018). Promoting diversity in the clinical and translational research workforce. *Journal of the National Medical Association, 110*(6), 598–605. https://doi.org/10.1016/j.jnma.2018.03.010

Faucett, E. A., Brenner, M. J., Thompson, D. M., & Flanary, V. A. (2022). Tackling the minority tax: A roadmap to redistributing engagement in diversity, equity, and inclusion initiatives. *Otolaryngology—Head and Neck Surgery, 166*(6), 1174–1181. https://doi.org/10.1177/01945998221091696

Fernández, M., Wheeler, D., & Alfonso, S. (2016). Embedding HIV mentoring programs in HIV research networks. *AIDS & Behavior, 20*, 281–287. https://doi.org/10.1007/s10461-016-1367-0

Fernandez, S. B., Clarke, R. D., Sheehan, D. M., Trepka, M. J., & Rose, S. M. (2021). Perceptual facilitators for and barriers to career progression: A qualitative study with female early stage investigators in health sciences. *Academic Medicine: Journal of the Association of American Medical Colleges, 96*(4), 576–584. https://doi.org/10.1097/ACM.0000000000003902

Flores, G., Mendoza, F. S., DeBaun, M. R., Fuentes-Afflick, E., Jones, V. F., Mendoza, J. A., Raphael, J. L., & Wang, C. J. (2019). Keys to academic success for underrepresented minority young investigators: Recommendations from the Research in Academic Pediatrics Initiative on Diversity (RAPID) National Advisory Committee. *International Journal for Equity in Health, 18*(1), 93. https://doi.org/10.1186/s12939-019-0995-1

Flores, G., Mendoza, F. S., Fuentes-Afflick, E., Mendoza, J. A., Pachter, L., Espinoza, J., Fernandez, C. R., Arnold, D. D. P., Brown, N. M., Gonzalez, K. M., Lopez, C., Owen, M. C., Parks, K. M., Reynolds, K. L., & Russell, C. J. (2016). Hot topics, urgent priorities, and ensuring success for racial/ethnic minority young investigators in academic pediatrics. *International Journal for Equity in Health, 15*(1), 201. https://doi.org/10.1186/s12939-016-0494-6

Forscher, P. S., Cox, W. T. L., Brauer, M., & Devine, P. G. (2019). Little race or gender bias in an experiment of initial review of NIH R01 grant proposals. *Nature Human Behaviour, 3*(3), 257–264. https://doi.org/10.1038/s41562-018-0517-y

Frogner, B. K. (2018). Update on the stock and supply of health services researchers in the united states. *Health Services Research, 53*(Suppl 2), 3945–3966. https://doi.org/10.1111/1475-6773.12988

Frogner, B. K. (2022). How the health services research workforce supply in the United States is evolving. *Health Services Research, 57*(2), 364–373. https://doi.org/10.1111/1475-6773.13934

Fuchs, J., Kouyate, A., Kroboth, L., & McFarland, W. (2016). Growing the pipeline of diverse HIV investigators: The impact of mentored research experiences to engage underrepresented minority students. *AIDS & Behavior, 20*, 249–257. https://doi.org/10.1007/s10461-016-1392-z

Gandhi, M., Fernandez, A., Stoff, D. M., Narahari, S., Blank, M., Fuchs, J., Evans, C. H., Kahn, J. S., & Johnson, M. O. (2014). Development and implementation of a workshop to enhance the effectiveness of mentors working with diverse mentees in HIV research. *AIDS Research and Human Retroviruses, 30*(8), 730–737. https://doi.org/10.1089/aid.2014.0018

Gandhi, M., & Johnson, M. (2016). Creating more effective mentors: Mentoring the mentor. *AIDS & Behavior, 20*, 294–303. https://doi.org/10.1007/s10461-016-1364-3

Ghaffarzadegan, N., Hawley, J., & Desai, A. (2014). Research workforce diversity: The case of balancing national versus international postdocs in us biomedical research. *Systems Research and Behavioral Science*, *31*(2), 301–315.

Ghaffarzadegan, N., Hawley, J., Larson, R., & Xue, Y. (2015). A note on PhD population growth in biomedical sciences: PhD population growth. *Systems Research and Behavioral Science*, *32*(3), 402–405. https://doi.org/10.1002/sres.2324

Gibbs, K. D., Basson, J., Xierali, I. M., & Broniatowski, D. A. (2016). Decoupling of the minority PhD talent pool and assistant professor hiring in medical school basic science departments in the US. *ELife*, *5*, e21393. https://doi.org/10.7554/eLife.21393

Gibbs, K. D., McGready, J., Bennett, J. C., & Griffin, K. (2014). Biomedical science Ph.D. career interest patterns by race/ethnicity and gender. *PLoS ONE*, *9*(12), e114736. https://doi.org/10.1371/journal.pone.0114736

Ginther, D. K., Kahn, S., & Schaffer, W. T. (2016). Gender, race/ethnicity, and National Institutes of Health R01 research awards: is there evidence of a double bind for women of color? *Academic Medicine*, *91*(8), 1098–1107. https://doi.org/10.1097/ACM.0000000000001278

Guillaume, R. O., & Apodaca, E. C. (2022). Early career faculty of color and promotion and tenure: The intersection of advancement in the academy and cultural taxation. *Race Ethnicity and Education*, *25*(4), 546–563. https://doi.org/10.1080/13613324.2020.1718084

Hamilton, N., & Haozous, E. A. (2017). Retention of faculty of color in academic nursing. *Nursing Outlook*, *65*(2), 212–221. https://doi.org/10.1016/j.outlook.2016.11.003

Harawa, N. T., Manson, S. M., Mangione, C. M., Penner, L. A., Norris, K. C., DeCarli, C., Scarinci, I. C., Zissimopoulos, J., Buchwald, D. S., Hinton, L., & Pérez-Stable, E. J. (2017). Strategies for enhancing research in aging health disparities by mentoring diverse investigators. *Journal of Clinical and Translational Science*, *1*(3), 167–175. https://doi.org/10.1017/cts.2016.23

Hardeman, R. R., Murphy, K. A., Karbeah, J., & Kozhimannil, K. B. (2018). Naming institutionalized racism in the public health literature: A systematic literature review. *Public Health Reports*, *133*(3), 240–249. https://doi.org/10.1177/0033354918760574

Heggeness, M. L., Evans, L., Pohlhaus, J. R., & Mills, S. L. (2016). Measuring diversity of the National Institutes of Health-funded workforce. *Academic Medicine: Journal of the Association of American Medical Colleges*, *91*(8), 1164–1172. https://doi.org/10.1097/ACM.0000000000001209

Hill, K. A., Desai, M. M., Chaudhry, S. I., Fancher, T., Nguyen, M., Wang, K., & Boatright, D. (2023). National Institutes of Health Diversity Supplement Awards by Medical School. *Journal of General Internal Medicine*, *38*(5), 1175–1179. https://doi.org/10.1007/s11606-022-07849-y

Hoff, K. A., Chu, C., Einarsdóttir, S., Briley, D. A., Hanna, A., & Rounds, J. (2022). Adolescent vocational interests predict early career success: Two 12-year longitudinal studies. *Applied Psychology*, *71*(1), 49–75. https://doi.org/10.1111/apps.12311

Holmes, A. G. D. (2020). Researcher Positionality—A Consideration of Its Influence and Place in Qualitative Research—A New Researcher Guide. *Shanlax International Journal of Education*, *8*(4), 1–10. https://doi.org/10.34293/education.v8i4.3232

Hoppe, T. A., Litovitz, A., Willis, K. A., Meseroll, R. A., Perkins, M. J., Hutchins, B. I., Davis, A. F., Lauer, M. S., Valantine, H. A., Anderson, J. M., & Santangelo, G. M. (2019). Topic choice contributes to the lower rate of NIH awards to African-American/black scientists. *Science Advances*, *5*(10), eaaw7238. https://doi.org/10.1126/sciadv.aaw7238

Howell, L. P., Wahl, S., Ryan, J., Gandour-Edwards, R., & Green, R..(2019). Educational and career development outcomes among undergraduate summer research interns: A pipeline for pathology, laboratory medicine, and biomedical science. *Academic Pathology*, *6*, 2374289519893105. https://doi.org/10.1177/2374289519893105

Huerta, J. J., Figuracion, M. T., Vazquez-Cortes, A., Hanna, R. R., Hernandez, A. C., Benitez, S. B., Sipelii, M. N., Brooks, T. C., ZuZero, D. T., Iopu, F. M. R. V., Romero, C. R., Chavez, A., Zell, A., Shugerman, S. R., Shannon, J. S., & Marriott, L. K. (2022). Interprofessional near-peer mentoring teams enhance cancer research training: Sustainable approaches for biomedical workforce development of historically underrepresented students. *The Journal of STEM Outreach*, *5*(2), 1–14. https://doi.org/10.15695/jstem/v5i2.10

Jean-Louis, G., Ayappa, I., Rapoport, D., Zizi, F., Airhihenbuwa, C., Okuyemi, K., & Ogedegbe, G. (2016). Mentoring junior URM scientists to engage in sleep health disparities research: Experience of the NYU PRIDE Institute. *Sleep Medicine*, *18*, 108–117. https://doi.org/10.1016/j.sleep.2015.09.010

Jeske, M., Vasquez, E., Fullerton, S. M., Saperstein, A., Bentz, M., Foti, N., Shim, J. K., & Lee, S. S.-J. (2022). Beyond inclusion: Enacting team equity in precision medicine research. *PloS One*, *17*(2), e0263750. https://doi.org/10.1371/journal.pone.0263750

Johnson, M. O., & Gandhi, M. (2015). A mentor training program improves mentoring competency for researchers working with early-career investigators from underrepresented backgrounds. *Advances in Health Sciences Education*, *20*(3), 683–689. https://doi.org/10.1007/s10459-014-9555-z

Jones, H. P., Vishwanatha, J. K., Yorio, T., & He, J. (2020). Preparing the next generation of diverse biomedical researchers: The University of North Texas Health Science Center's Initiative for Maximizing Student Development (IMSD) predoctoral program. *Ethnicity & Disease*, *30*(1), 65–74. https://doi.org/10.18865/ed.30.1.65

Julion, W., Reed, M., Bounds, D. T., Cothran, F., Gamboa, C., & Sumo, J. (2019). A group think tank as a discourse coalition to promote minority nursing faculty retention. *Nursing*

Outlook, *67*(5), 586–595. https://doi.org/10.1016/j.outlook.2019.03.003

Kaatz, A., Lee, Y.-G., Potvien, A., Magua, W., Filut, A., Bhattacharya, A., Leatherberry, R., Zhu, X., & Carnes, M. (2016). Analysis of National Institutes of Health R01 application critiques, impact, and criteria scores: Does the sex of the Principal Investigator make a difference? *Academic Medicine*, *91*(8), 1080–1088. https://doi.org/10.1097/ACM.0000000000001272

Kameny, R. R., DeRosier, M. E., Taylor, L. C., McMillen, J. S., Knowles, M. M., & Pifer, K. (2014). Barriers to career success for minority researchers in the behavioral sciences. *Journal of Career Development*, *41*(1), 43–61. https://doi.org/10.1177/0894845312472254

Kippenbrock, T., & Emory, J. (2021). National Institute of Nursing Research grant funding recipients: Hispanic and nurses of color are lagging. *Hispanic Health Care International*, *19*(3), 203–206. https://doi.org/10.1177/1540415321998722

Krieger, N., Boyd, R. W., Maio, F. D., & Maybank, A. (2021). Medicine's privileged gatekeepers: Producing harmful ignorance about racism and health [blog]. *Health Affairs Forefront*. https://doi.org/10.1377/forefront.20210415.305480

Liu, F., Holme, P., Chiesa, M., AlShebli, B., & Rahwan, T. (2023). Gender inequality and self-publication are common among academic editors. *Nature Human Behaviour*, *7*(3), Article 3. https://doi.org/10.1038/s41562-022-01498-1

López, A. M., Rodríguez, J. E., Browning Hawes, K., Marsden, A., Ayer, D., Ziegenfuss, D. H., & Okuyemi, K. (2021). Preparing historically underrepresented trainees for biomedical cancer research careers at Huntsman Cancer Institute/University of Utah Health. *Medical Education Online*, *26*(1), 1929045. https://doi.org/10.1080/10872981.2021.1929045

Marriott, L. K., Raz Link, A., Anitori, R. P., Blackwell, E. A., Blas, A., Brock, J., Burke, T. K., Burrows, J. A., Cabrera, A. P., Helsham, D., Liban, L. B., Mackiewicz, M. R., Maruyama, M., Milligan-Myhre, K. C. A., Panelinan, P. J. C., Hattori-Uchima, M., Reed, R., Simon, B. E., Solomon, B., . . . ,

& Crespo, C. J. (2021). Supporting bio-medical research training for historically underrepresented undergraduates using interprofessional, nonformal education structures. *Journal of the Scholarship of Teaching and Learning, 21*(1), 241–286. https://doi.org/10.14434/josotl.v21i1.30430

Marriott, L. K., Shugerman, S. R., Chavez, A., Crocker Daniel, L., Martinez, A., Zebroski, D. J., Mishalanie, S., Zell, A., Dest, A., Pozhidayeva, D., Wenzel, E. S., Omotoy, H. L., Druker, B. J., & Shannon, J. (2022). Knight Scholars Program: A tiered three-year mentored training program for urban and rural high school students Increases interest and self-efficacy in interprofessional cancer research. *Journal of STEM Outreach, 5*(2), 1–16. https://doi.org/10.15695/jstem/v5i2.06

Merchant, R. M., Del Rio, C., & Boulware, L. E. (2021). Structural racism and scientific journals—A teachable moment. *JAMA, 326*(7), 607. https://doi.org/10.1001/jama.2021.12105

Moceri, J. T. (2022). Overview and summary: Racism and nursing: diverse perspectives. *OJIN: The Online Journal of Issues in Nursing, 27*(1), Overview and Summary. https://doi.org/10.3912/OJIN.Vol27No01ManOS

Moore, C. L., Wang, N., Davis, D., Aref, F., Manyibe, E. O., Washington, A. L., Johnson, J., Eugene-Cross, K., Muhammad, A., & Jennings-Jones, D. (2017). Key informant perspectives on federal research agency policy and systems and scientific workforce diversity development: a companion study. *Rehabilitation Research, Policy & Education, 31*(3), 230–252. https://doi.org/10.1891/2168-6653.31.3.230

National Academies of Sciences, Engineering, and Medicine. (2017). *2016 Year in Review: Roundtable on Population Health Improvement*. Washington, DC: The National Academies Press. https://doi.org/10.17226/27078

National Academies of Sciences, Engineering, and Medicine. (2021). *The future of nursing 2020–2030: charting a path to achieve health equity*, (pp. 25982). National Academies Press. https://doi.org/10.17226/25982

National Commission to Address Racism in Nursing. (2021). *Racism in Nursing*. American Nurses Association. https://www.nursingworld.org/~49c4d0/globalassets/practiceandpolicy/workforce/commission-to-address-racism/racism-in-nursing-report-series.pdf

National Institutes of Health. (2022, August 15). *Racial Disparities in NIH Funding. SWD at NIH* [Governmental]. U.S. Department of Health & Human Services. https://diversity.nih.gov/building-evidence/racial-disparities-nih-funding

National Library of Medicine. (2023, August 15). *PubMed Overview* [Governmental]. National Library of Medicine. https://pubmed.ncbi.nlm.nih.gov/about/

Norris, K. C., McCreath, H. E., Hueffer, K., Aley, S. B., Chavira, G., Christie, C. A., Crespi, C. M., Crespo, C., D'Amour, G., Eagan, K., Echegoyen, L. E., Feig, A., Foroozesh, M., Guerrero, L. R., Johanson, K., Kamangar, F., Kingsford, L., LaCourse, W., Maccalla, N. M.-G., ... Seeman, T. (2020). Baseline characteristics of the 2015–2019 first year student cohorts of the NIH Building Infrastructure Leading to Diversity (BUILD) program. *Ethnicity & Disease, 30*(4), 681–692. https://doi.org/10.18865/ed.30.4.681

Ofili, E. O., Tchounwou, P. B., Fernandez-Repollet, E., Yanagihara, R., Akintobi, T. H., Lee, J. E., Malouhi, M., Garner, S. T., Jr., Hayes, T. T., Baker, A. R., Dent, A. L., 2nd, Abdelrahim, M., Rollins, L., Chang, S. P., Sy, A., Hernandez, B. Y., Bullard, P. L., Noel, R. J., Jr., Shiramizu, B., ... Norris, K. C. (2019). The Research Centers in Minority Institutions (RCMI) Translational Research Network: Building and sustaining capacity for multi-site basic biomedical, clinical and behavioral research. *Ethnicity & Disease, 29*(Suppl 1), 135–144. https://doi.org/10.18865/ed.29.S1.135

Olukotun, O., Mkandawire, E., Antilla, J., Alfaifa, F., Weitzel, J., Scheer, V., Olukotun, M., & Mkandawire-Valhmu, L. (2021). An analysis of reflections on researcher positionality. *The Qualitative Report, 26*(5), 1411–1426. https://doi.org/10.46743/2160-3715/2021.4613

Oncology Nursing Society. (2021, September 9). *Nursing has a long history of racism. Now Is the time to overcome it.* https://voice.ons.org/conferences/nursing-has-a-long-history-of-racism-now-is-the-time-to-overcome-it

Richardson, D. M., Keller, T. E., Wolf, D. S. S., Zell, A., Morris, C., & Crespo, C. J. (2017). BUILD EXITO: a multi-level intervention to support diversity in health-focused research. *BMC Proceedings*, *11*(S12), 19. https://doi.org/10.1186/s12919-017-0080-y

Rivers, R., Norris, K. C., Hui, G., Halpern-Felsher, B., Dodge-Francis, C., Guerrero, L. R., Golshan, A., Brinkley, K., Tran, K., McLaughlin, S., Antolin, N., Yoshida, T., Caffey-Fleming, D. E., & Agodoa, L. (2020). The NIDDK high school short-term research experience for underrepresented persons. *Ethnicity & Disease*, *30*(1), 5–14. https://doi.org/10.18865/ed.30.1.5

Rollins, G. (2022). Racism in nursing: the latest report. *American Nurse*. https://www.myamericannurse.com/reporting-on-racism-in-nursing/

Rubio, D. M., Hamm, M. E., Mayowski, C. A., Nouraie, S. M., Quarshie, A., Seto, T., Shaheen, M., Soto De Laurido, L. E., & Norman, M. K. (2019). Developing a training program to diversify the biomedical research workforce. *Academic Medicine*, *94*(8), 1115–1121. https://doi.org/10.1097/ACM.0000000000002654

Rubio, D. M., Mayowski, C. A., & Norman, M. K. (2018). A multi-pronged approach to diversifying the workforce. *International Journal of Environmental Research and Public Health*, *15*(10), 2219. https://doi.org/10.3390/ijerph15102219

Salazar, J. W., Claytor, J. D., Habib, A. R., Guduguntla, V., & Redberg, R. F. (2021). Gender, race, ethnicity, and sexual orientation of editors at leading medical and scientific journals: a cross-sectional survey. *JAMA Internal Medicine*, *181*(9), 1248–1251. https://doi.org/10.1001/jamainternmed.2021.2363

Salter, P. S., & Haugen, A. D. (2017). Critical race studies in psychology. In B.Gough (Ed.), *The Palgrave handbook of critical social psychology*. Palgrave Macmillan UK. https://doi.org/10.1057/978-1-137-51018-1_7

Shahram, S. Z. (2023). Five ways 'health scholars' are complicit in upholding health inequities, and how to stop. *International Journal for Equity in Health*, *22*(1), 15. https://doi.org/10.1186/s12939-022-01763-9

Shihabuddin, B. S., Fritter, J., Ellison, A. M., & Cruz, A. T. (2022). Diversity among research coordinators in a pediatric emergency medicine research collaborative network. *Journal of Clinical and Translational Science*, *7*(1), e46. https://doi.org/10.1017/cts.2022.448

Smalley, K. B., & Warren, J. C. (2020). Disparities Elimination Summer Research Experience (DESRE): An intensive summer research training program to promote diversity in the biomedical research workforce. *Ethnicity & Disease*, *30*(1), 47–54. https://doi.org/10.18865/ed.30.1.47

Smiley, R. A., Ruttinger, C., Oliveira, C. M., Hudson, L. R., Allgeyer, R., Reneau, K. A., Silvestre, J. H., & Alexander, M. (2021). The 2020 national nursing workforce survey. *Journal of Nursing Regulation*, *12*(1), S1–S96.

Sopher, C. J., Adamson, B. J. S., Andrasik, M. P., Flood, D. M., Wakefield, S. F., Stoff, D. M., Cook, R. S., Kublin, J. G., & Fuchs, J. D. (2015). Enhancing diversity in the public health research workforce: The research and mentorship program for future HIV vaccine scientists. *American Journal of Public Health*, *105*(4), 823–830. https://doi.org/10.2105/AJPH.2014.302076

Tagge, R., Lackland, D. T., & Ovbiagele, B. (2021). The TRANSCENDS program: Rationale and overview. *Journal of the Neurological Sciences*, *420*, 117218. https://doi.org/10.1016/j.jns.2020.117218

Thakar, M. S., Mitchell-Miland, C., Morone, N. E., Althouse, A. D., Murrell, A. J., Rubio, D. M., & White, G. E. (2023). Perseverance and consistency of interest in underrepresented post-doctoral fellows and early-career faculty. *Journal of Clinical and Translational Science*, *7*(1), e100. https://doi.org/10.1017/cts.2023.523

Thoman, D. B., Brown, E. R., Mason, A. Z., Harmsen, A. G., & Smith, J. L. (2015). The role of altruistic values in motivating underrepresented minority students for biomedicine. *BioScience, 65*(2), 183–188. https://doi.org/10.1093/biosci/biu199

Thorpe, R. J., Jr., Vishwanatha, J. K., Harwood, E. M., Krug, E. L., Unold, T., Eide Boman, K., & Jones, H. P. (2020). The impact of grantsmanship self-efficacy on early stage investigators of the national research mentoring network steps toward academic research. *Ethnicity & Disease, 30*(1), 75–82. https://doi.org/10.18865/ed.30.1.75

Ullah, R., Asghar, I., & Griffiths, M. G. (2023). An integrated methodology for bibliometric analysis: A case study of internet of things in healthcare applications. *Sensors, 23*(1), 67. https://doi.org/10.3390/s23010067

Urizar, G. G., Henriques, L., Chun, C.-A., Buonora, P., Vu, K.-P. L., Galvez, G., & Kingsford, L. (2017). Advancing research opportunities and promoting pathways in graduate education: A systemic approach to BUILD training at California State University, Long Beach (CSULB). *BMC Proceedings, 11*(S12), 26. https://doi.org/10.1186/s12919-017-0088-3

Vishwanatha, J. K., Basha, R., Nair, M., & Jones, H. P. (2019). An institutional coordinated plan for effective partnerships to achieve health equity and biomedical workforce diversity. *Ethnicity & Disease, 29*(Suppl 1), 129–134. https://doi.org/10.18865/ed.29.S1.129

Wiley, K., Dixon, B. E., Grannis, S. J., & Menachemi, N. (2020). Underrepresented racial minorities in biomedical informatics doctoral programs: Graduation trends and academic placement (2002–2017). *Journal of the American Medical Informatics Association, 27*(11), 1641–1647. https://doi.org/10.1093/jamia/ocaa206

Williams, D. R., Lawrence, J. A., & Davis, B. A. (2019). Racism and health: evidence and needed research. *Annual Review of Public Health, 40*(1), 105–125. https://doi.org/10.1146/annurev-publhealth-040218-043750

Williams, S. N., Thakore, B. K., & McGee, R. (2016). Coaching to augment mentoring to achieve faculty diversity: A randomized controlled trial. *Academic Medicine, 91*(8), 1128–1135. https://doi.org/10.1097/ACM.0000000000001026

Yoon, S., Falzon, L., Anderson, N. B., & Davidson, K. W. (2019). A look at the increasing demographic representation within behavioral medicine. *Journal of Behavioral Medicine, 42*(1), 57–66. https://doi.org/10.1007/s10865-018-9983-y

Zambrana, R. E., & Williams, D. R. (2022). The intellectual roots of current knowledge on racism and health: Relevance to policy and the national equity discourse. *Health Affairs, 41*(2), 163–170. https://doi.org/10.1377/hlthaff.2021.01439

Zhou, C., Okafor, C., Hagood, J., & DeLisser, H. M. (2021). Penn Access Summer Scholars program: A mixed method analysis of a virtual offering of a premedical diversity summer enrichment program. *Medical Education Online, 26*(1), 1905918. https://doi.org/10.1080/10872981.2021.1905918

Zupic, I., & Čater, T. (2015). Bibliometric methods in management and organization. *Organizational Research Methods, 18*(3), 429–472. https://doi.org/10.1177/1094428114562629

5

Administration and Leadership: Policy, Advocacy, Clinical Practice, and Academia

Deborah Finn-Romero, DNP, RN, PHN, PACT
Melissa Hinds, MSN, RN

INTRODUCTION

This chapter focuses on the development and implementation of policies within health care infrastructures. It explores the roles of nurses and health care professionals as legislative policy advocates, clinical practice leaders, and academic administrators engaged in creating and leveraging policies related to social and structural determinants of health (SSDH). It also delves into the active participation of health care institutional leaders in driving infrastructural changes toward achieving health equity. The purpose of this chapter is to provide resources and inspiration to leaders who seek to advance their institutions in promoting health equity through the formation and implementation of policies and procedures. Essential considerations in this process encompass addressing discrimination—both implicit and explicit bias—harnessing the power of research and making informed decisions about policy development and its effective implementation.

Values and Alignment

Leaders have responsibility to organizations and community members to envision and set the path forward to an equitable future for all. As members of the National League for NLN/Walden University College of Nursing Institute for Social Determinants of Health and Social Change, each of us commit to the work of advocacy, creating and supporting policies of equity and social justice. We call on all administrators and leaders to join this crucial work of recreating our structures through the lens of Social and Structural Determinants of Health, laying the groundwork for success for future generations that follow in our footsteps.

Chapter Objectives

Upon completion of this chapter, the learner will be able to:

1. Understand the role of health care professionals as policy advocates.
2. Examine leadership strategies for achieving health equity.
3. Recognize the impact of bias and discrimination in health care.
4. Leverage research for evidence-based policy development.

BACKGROUND

Policies drive administrative changes; therefore, the transformation of educational and practice institutions into entities that reflect the principles of SSDH occurs through the integration of policy changes. Developing and implementing operational policies and practices, such as implicit bias training, cultural humility programs, and awareness training regarding microaggressions for all staff and faculty, are essential steps in the process of reshaping the institutional culture. This transformation involves recognizing and addressing health inequities within the institution's systems, while also modeling advocacy participation in broader social change.

The duty of health care providers extends beyond settings like hospitals and primary care facilities. In the increasingly complex American society, meeting the health needs of our populations has grown equally intricate, necessitating a deep dive into community structures. Governments at all levels—city, county, state, and federal—are confronted with challenges related to health care costs, uninsured patients, limited resources for public transportation to care providers and pharmacies, declining educational accomplishments affecting health literacy, food deserts in redlined neighborhoods, and various other issues impacting health.

STRATEGIES TO INTEGRATE SSDH NEED INTO ADMINISTRATIVE POLICY

Nursing administration must demonstrate a commitment to identifying resource gaps, including funding and content expertise, as a crucial initial step in improving SSDH. Additionally, measures must be taken to locate, secure, and provide the necessary resources for nursing and interprofessional development. Both current and emerging nurse leaders should serve as role models by exhibiting skills that are culturally responsive, equity-centric, and advocacy-minded.

Governments, nongovernmental organizations (NGOs), and major health care organizations are increasingly recognizing the need to address the broader societal issues, including racism, as a pivotal step toward improving health outcomes. The federal government's Office of Health Promotion and Disease Prevention (OHPDP) is a division of the U.S. Department of Health and Human Services (USDHHS). This office's mission is to lead the nation in health improvement by establishing and promoting health priorities, translating science into policy, providing essential tools, improving health literacy, and working toward equitable access to health care (USDHHS, 2022). Through OHPDP, the establishment of Healthy People measurable 10-year objectives began in 1990. Every decade since, Healthy People establishes the health priorities of the nation. Healthy People 2030 features the SSDH framework, which outlines the mission, vision, foundational principles, overarching goals, and plan of action (NASEM, 2019; Office of Health Promotion and Illness Prevention. Healthy People 2030, n.d.).

The SSDH framework serves as the foundation for discussion, targeted changes, and progress evaluation within American society through *Healthy People 2030*. Within *Healthy People 2030*, the "Leading Indicators" and "Health Objectives" serve as benchmarks for the health of the American population (Office of Health Promotion and Illness Prevention. Healthy People 2030, n.d.). As of this publication date, *Healthy People 2030* allows for searches based on specific populations, including Adolescents, Children, Infants, LGBT, Men, Older Adults, People with Disabilities, Parents or Caregivers, Women, and the Workforce. However, it is worth noting that historically excluded and underrepresented populations, such as Black or Indigenous communities, are not explicitly mentioned within these categories. Instead, monitoring and addressing health status and needs of underrepresented populations, including racial underrepresented groups, are the responsibility of the Office of Minority Health within the United States Department of Health and Human Services (U.S. Department of Health and Human Services, Office of Minority Health, [n.d]).

Efforts to enhance understanding of SSDH extend to nursing educational institutions. On the basis of growing evidence of the relationship between SSDH and implicit bias negatively impacting health outcomes (Jackson et al., 2023; Macias-Konstantopoulos et al., 2023), nursing programs nationwide are actively taking steps to address issues of implicit bias within organizational policies and practices. These steps include the provision of implicit bias training for faculty and staff and the integration of implicit bias training into the curriculum. Nursing program administrators and faculty are beginning to embrace self-assessment and are evolving to align with the new paradigm of socially conscious health care. As noted by Batra et al. (2022), there is room for improvement in nursing academic programs when it comes to advancing social missions, such as addressing racism, fostering community, and participating in political engagement. Activities related to program self-awareness, equitable admission practices, and the development of meaningful curricula pertaining to SSDH are essential for the future of nursing (Zappas et al., 2021). Nursing programs across the nation are called to actively review, test, and implement internal policies and processes, including admission criteria and holistic applications, in pursuit of these goals.

Health care institutional policies and practices must be examined through the lens of SSDH. Leadership support for practices addressing SSDH is paramount for enhancing health outcomes. Notably, Medicare rules that offer financial incentives to prevent readmissions for the same conditions have proven unsuccessful (Banerjee et al., 2021), underscoring the need to implement alternative preventative measures. In this context, considerations such as racism and SSDH must be integrated into the process of policy formation. As highlighted by Rambachan et al. (2022), when controlling for SSDH factors, people of color experienced higher rates of hospital readmission.

GOVERNMENT POLICY FORMATION AND ADVOCACY

U.S. governments are increasingly recognizing the necessity for change to improve health outcomes (National Institutes of Health, 2023; Office of Health Promotion and

Illness Prevention, 2022). However, change within large systems tends to be slow. Often, the identification of critical issues begins at grassroots levels. Raising awareness about unmet needs and their impacts on communities requires targeted advocacy. This advocacy involves engaging with leaders, presenting data that represents concerns, and proposing real-world solutions. Although our governments are responsible for establishing and leading priorities within specific jurisdictions, health care providers recognize no such boundaries. In fact, it is the duty of every caregiver to advocate for the health and well-being of any individual under their care. Health care providers and educators are poised to champion the needs of the community at governmental and executive levels, both through research and advocacy efforts.

Advocacy

Since the 1980s, nursing leaders have actively engaged in shaping social policy (Fyfee, 2009; Roper et al., 1992). In order to raise awareness on public health issues and underscore the profound impact of economic, political, social, and cultural factors in relation to health (Lewenson, 1996), nurses began participating in the political process and advocating for policy formation and change. The National League for Nursing (NLN) operates at the national level, advocating for public policies aimed at addressing health inequities. The NLN 2023/2024 Public Policy Agenda underscores that the top priorities in nursing and public policy must revolve around education, access, workforce, and diversity National League for Nursing (NLN). (2024). The values of SSDH have been an integral part of the NLN's history, dating back to 1953 with the position statement, "All activities of the NLN shall include all groups regardless of race, color, religion and sex." Additionally, in 1959, the *Patient Bill of Rights* emphasized that "Nursing personnel respect the individuality, dignity, and rights of every person regardless of race, color, creed, national origin, social or economic status" (NLN, n.d.). The NLN remains committed to championing SSDH issues through initiatives such as Taking Aim (NLN, 2021) and the NLN/Walden Institute for Social Determinants of Health and Social Change (NLN/Walden University, n.d.). These endeavors play a significant role in shaping the United States' approach to health care through advocacy efforts, as well as contribution to the *Future of Nursing* reports (National Academy of Sciences, Engineering, and Sciences [NASEM], 2021).

Nurses are increasingly recognized as a potent force for health care reform, often working through organizations and adopting an interprofessional approach. The Patient Protection and Affordable Care Act (2010) marked a significant milestone by expanding nursing education, promoting advanced nursing practice, and fostering leadership development. This expansion has led to a surge in nurses assuming leadership positions within health care organizations, governmental bodies, and policymaking groups (Cleveland et al., 2019). Although these advancements acknowledge the influential role nurses play in health care, there remains substantial work to be done, particularly in addressing SSDH specifically. As emphasized in the *Future of Nursing* (NASEM, 2021) report, it is imperative to strengthen nursing education by addressing SSDH to advance health equity.

To drive substantial societal changes and enhance health outcomes for all American populations, thought leaders and elected officials must expedite the identification and transformation of issues that adversely affect the nation. Achieving this objective requires the engagement of experts who can bring pressing concerns to the forefront for review. Such a process involves rigorous research, advocacy efforts, and collaborative partnerships. According to Fuller (2016), bioethicists and health care providers must actively engage in advocacy and activism to challenge the prevailing status quo. Furthermore, professional organizations play a pivotal role in advocacy efforts, which are indispensable for effecting lasting change, particularly in addressing racism as a root cause of health inequity.

Research Support

Research focusing on SSHD categories and related issues plays a crucial role in justifying policy and legislative changes. A glaring example of racial inequities exists in maternal and infant mortality rates. Black infants are 2.4 times more likely to die than their White counterparts (USDHHS, 2022). This disturbing trend reveals persistent and significantly elevated rates among non-White infants for over a century, despite an overall decrease in mortality rates for all racial groups since the 1980s (USDHHS, Office of Minority Health, 2022; Singh & Yu, 2019). Conclusions drawn from research emphasize the urgent need for stronger social integration of racial groups at a regional level, increased public financial investment in health services programs, and comprehensive efforts to address the pervasive inequities experienced by Black individuals in America (Kandasamy et al., 2020). Furthermore, a separate study revealed that approximately half of medical providers held misconceptions about Black populations, such as believing they had higher pain tolerance and thicker skin (Hoffman et al., 2016). These revelations prompted the State of California to take legislative action in 2019 by mandating implicit bias training for all nurses. The goal was to enhance maternal and newborn care and improve outcomes for patients. Subsequently, in January 2023, all prelicensure nursing schools were mandated to provide comprehensive implicit bias training to their students. Following suit, the State of Michigan implemented similar regulations in 2022.

SOCIAL AND STRUCTURAL DETERMINANTS OF HEALTH IN CLINICAL POLICY AND PRACTICE

Increasingly, health care systems are recognizing structural determinants as root causes of societal and health inequities. Patients' experiences, such as discrimination, poverty, limited access to health care, trauma, involvement with the criminal justice system, and housing instability, highlight the need for health care support services (Bay Area Regional Health Inequities Initiative, 2015). It is crucial for institutions to establish policies that specifically address the impact of SSDH on patients.

Resources and Funding

Administrative philosophies that embrace the development of partnerships with community agencies for essential service can enhance health outcomes. Supportive nurse leadership can play a central role in addressing SSDH, advancing health equity, and ultimately improving health outcomes (Lathrop, 2013). Nursing administration must establish and implement policies that empower clinical nurse educators to tackle these inequities by threading SSDH-related content into nursing training. Training reflecting health equity and SSDH needs to be included in new orientation, annual skill development, hands-on experience with experienced staff, and engagement in interprofessional activities.

Educational and Leadership Investment

Committed and engaged leadership is central to transforming organizations and sustaining change (Doherty et al., 2022). Clinical administrative leaders should prioritize educating themselves about SSDH to advance health equity. Committed and engaged leadership starts with self. Leaders for social change must take time with themselves. Commitment starts with time invested in knowing yourself first—your ideals, values, and motivation for taking on the work of eliminating social and health inequities. Next, it involves the development of a critical consciousness, or the ability to identify, critique, and challenge sociopolitical forces that produce inequity (Jemal, 2017). The crux of critical consciousness is learning how to recognize social, political, and economic contradictions (Jemal, 2017).

Nurse leaders can become trailblazers in initiating this transformation of care. Leaders who can effectively model communication about SSDH care needs may have a significant impact on staff transformation and the implementation of SSDH into practice. Establishing a communication infrastructure through continued education and staff development can inform and influence health-related decisions and actions while addressing SSDH (Goulbourne & Yanovitzky, 2021).

Administrators can implement strategies to support the integration of SSDH-centered care, including investing in the collection and evaluation of patient data that may identify race-based inequities. Data allows leadership to identify policy and program interventions to correct identified inequities. In addition, it helps nurses in administrative or leadership positions gain critical self-awareness about racial inequities in their organizations (Nardi et al., 2020). Nurse leaders working toward racial equity can use data to set and communicate priorities, foster organizational buy-in, and develop mechanisms that support accountability for focusing on SSDH. Health inequities occur within and outside of health care institutions. Use of data and critical self-reflection to consider that existing structural racism and oppression may be present within existing organizational policies and practices is a recommended practice.

Diversification of Workforce

Another essential aspect of addressing SSDH is cultivating a diverse workforce in various roles, which can help reduce health inequities and work toward health equity. A significant emphasis should be placed on developing diverse nursing leadership within health care provider organizations, including steering committees that create spaces for a wide range of experiences, voices, and perspectives. Nursing administration can proactively concentrate on establishing program initiatives to address the limited representation of diversity in the health care workforce, especially in areas where providers do not reflect the demographics of the communities they serve. To deliver high-quality and accessible care to patients and communities, nursing administration and leadership must advocate for a health care workforce that is representative of communities it serves and provide opportunities for staff to learn from, with, and about each other to enhance patient outcomes.

SOCIAL AND STRUCTURAL DETERMINANTS OF HEALTH IN CLINICAL POLICY AND PRACTICE: A CASE EXEMPLAR IN MENTAL HEALTH

Why Address the Social and Structural Determinants of Mental Health?

Social and structural determinants of health (SSDH) can influence health in positive and negative ways. Evidence demonstrates how income inequality, discrimination, adverse childhood experiences, food insecurity, and other adverse environmental exposures can lead to poor health and disproportionately poor health outcomes for certain population segments (Shim & Compton, 2018). Experiencing gaps in access to positive factors can harm a person's mental health care and act as both a risk factor for and a consequence of behavioral disorders. For example, discrimination, unemployment/underemployment, limited access to transportation, or inadequate health care negatively impacts the course and outcomes of an individual's behavioral disorder and comorbid physical illnesses (NIDA, 2022). Also, exposure to or experiencing adverse SSDH factors can negatively influence personal choices, living conditions, and opportunities and increase the level of stress experienced by individuals, which can then increase the risk of experiencing substance use problems and mental health issues (NIDA, 2022).

The need to address SSDH is even more notable, as research shows there is a shorter life expectancy between individuals with serious mental illness (SMI) or substance use disorder (SUD) of about 10 to 20 years than the general population, and many premature deaths are avoidable (de Mooij et al., 2019). Studies have also shown that metabolic, respiratory, and cardiovascular diseases (CVD) are the main physical illnesses in patients with SMI and are modifiable risk factors (Momen et al., 2022). SSDH can shape a person's likelihood of experiencing behavioral health and substance use issues, and also their ability to obtain treatment and maintain recovery. They can also improve early physical health screenings to identify medical diseases and lifestyle interventions to reduce the risk of premature death. In recent years, the New York State insurers, health care providers, and communities have been paying greater attention to SSDH and mental health. Fiscal, clinical, and public health priorities have driven the shifting focus on health equity and social justice considerations. Advancing health equity means working to ensure that every individual has the opportunity to be as healthy as possible. Although there is an increased awareness that improving health and attaining health equity requires broader approaches that address the social, economic, justice, and environmental factors that influence health, a significant gap exists in addressing SSDH through behavioral health strategies, policies, and programs.

SSDH are particularly impactful in historically excluded and underrepresented populations. Historically underserved, disadvantaged, and underrepresented populations suffer an extraordinary disease burden. Heightened exposure to social, economic, spatial (e.g., access/proximity to health care, age distribution, rurality, access to employment centers, and population density), and environmental risk factors contribute to population health inequities. These include high rates of adverse childhood experiences, disproportionate marketing and sales of tobacco and alcohol in specific communities (Lee et al., 2020; Ribisl et al., 2017), and inadequate access to education and employment opportunities. Depending on the geographic area, a historically underserved, disadvantaged, and underrepresented person living in New York may encounter environmental risk factors and a chronically under-resourced health care system, and experience the health impacts of intergenerational historical trauma (McKnight-Eily et al., 2021). In addition to the known impacts on physical health, several studies have highlighted various ways that SDH impacts mental health outcomes within specific populations. Unemployment, unstable employment, and the conditions in which the individual works have been linked to increased psychological distress (Pevalin et al., 2017). Lower incomes and financial strain or disadvantage can contribute to poor mental health and lead to self-harm, suicide attempts, and depression (Alegría et al., 2018).

New York State Behavioral Health Service Providers Call to Action

New York State has an extensive, multifaceted mental health system, serving more than 700,000 individuals annually (Office of Mental Health [OMH], n.d.). In addition to the many people who access services, the State's increasing diversity in residents, languages, and geography requires shifting service provision to meet the needs of care recipients. To meet this need, the New York State Office of Mental Health (OMH) addresses the mental health burden experienced by the population served through statewide influence on policy and practice and creates pipelines to increase the diversity of their workforce. OMH is explicitly working to eliminate disparities in access, quality, and treatment outcomes by addressing social determinants, experiences of discrimination, environmental stressors, economic hardship, and social support by providing educational guidance, consultation, and data-driven policy change.

Meeting the needs of New York State's diverse populations has been essential to changes in policies, procedures, and practices that have been integral to addressing disparities in the delivery of mental health services. As the State moves away from delivering services in traditional settings and working to engage people in their communities, service providers need to be knowledgeable of, identify, and address social determinants. Education can help providers to enhance their awareness of SDH and best practices. Providers need to continue to learn and increase their knowledge to understand how other factors, such as SSDH disparities, can and will impact outcomes.

Understanding the interrelationships among upstream, midstream, and downstream factors and interventions is necessary to fully comprehend and influence the health of individuals and communities. Upstream policy changes that promote population health and integrated social interventions are needed to connect individuals to social services, including healthy food, affordable housing, and transportation. However, providers need education, training, and support to engage robustly at all three levels. Below, we describe how the New York State OMH and the Center for Practice Innovations (CPI) address SSDH and social needs through upstream clinical policy and practice interventions.

"Upstream" Efforts at the New York State Office of Mental Health

In 2018, the New York State Office of Mental Health prioritized SDH as a vital knowledge area that providers must understand and address. As outlined in the document, *The Social Determinants of Mental Health: A White Paper Detailing Promising Practices and Opportunities at the New York State Office of Mental Health* (Rotter & Compton, 2020), the 25-member New York Statewide Multicultural Advisory Committee advises the New York State OMH on policy, programs, procedures, and activities addressing disparities in access, quality, and outcomes for members of historically underserved, disadvantaged, and underrepresented populations. Committee membership includes diverse consumers of mental health services, experts in the field, policymakers, and researchers. OMH, participating behavioral health agencies, and intermediary organizations actively worked to identify previous or existing internal activities which address SDH for the individuals to whom they provide services.

The OMH operates psychiatric centers across the State and regulates, certifies, and oversees over 4,500 local government and nonprofit agency-operated programs. In August 2018, the New York State (NYS) OMH established a Social Determinants of Mental Health (SDMH) Workgroup (Rotter & Compton, 2020). The role of the group was to help NYS OMH learn what efforts other state or city agencies had implemented to address SSDH and work to develop a social determinants agenda. The workgroup also used the social determinants framework (Solar & Irwin, 2010) to help guide efforts to prevent mental illnesses and substance use disorders in the community, address health disparities and inequities, and help frame and prioritize a focus on the social needs of existing clients. The framework illustrates the different types of SDMH and the relationship between these determinants and health, as well as helps prioritize policy interventions to address health care issues effectively and efficiently. The group identified eight areas of SDMH-related activities or spheres of influence (Box 5.1). The NYS OMH used each area of the sphere to frame its thinking on how it already addresses, proposed new initiatives, and identified potential opportunities for each sphere to provide higher-quality care, improve SDH and health outcomes, and work to reduce social and policy barriers.

BOX 5.1

The Office of Mental Health Spheres of Influence

Data Collection and Analysis
Funding
Informal Influence
Policy Making
Regulation and Licensing
Research
State Operations
Training

Source: Rotter, M., & Compton, M. T. (2020). *The Social determinants of mental health: A white paper detailing promising practices and opportunities at the New York State Office of Mental Health.* https://omh.ny.gov/omhweb/sdmh-white-paper.pdf

NYS OMH was already working to address SDMH as part of the agency's standards and areas of commitment. These needs arose within state-operated facilities when providers became aware of the social needs or social disadvantages among clients and worked to address them in various ways. Given the importance of social determinants on behavioral health outcomes and the OMH's influence on policy and program at the statewide and local levels, they began taking a more coordinated and intentional approach to addressing SDMH for both individuals they serve and the community.

Policymaking, regulations and licensing, training, and data collection and analysis are four of the eight identified SDMH-related activities areas that directly influence statewide clinical policy and practice. For example, OMH collaborated with the Department of Health to set Medicaid reimbursement policies for Managed Care Organizations (MCOs) that incorporate requirements for addressing SDH in value-based payment standards. New York requires value-based payment (VBP) contracting goals for MCOs, and the State ties financial incentives to meeting goals. MCOs must implement at least one SDH intervention within their contract (Daniel-Robinson & Moore, 2019). The requirement allows program reimbursement for education, employment, and peer support services. OMH also supports the implementation of the National CLAS (National Standard for Culturally and Linguistically Appropriate Services) Standards (USDHHS, 2016) into policies, standards of care, and regulation. The National CLAS Standards are validated measures that improve quality, advance health equity, and help eliminate health care disparities.

In contrast, the other domains focus on how OMH uses its influence to advance research, provide funding, implement changes in the state operation settings, and endorse activities that support addressing social determinants. For example, OMH provides initial or ongoing funding for diverse initiatives and research addressing social determinants. In clinical settings, OMH also addresses social needs and determinants (i.e., education, employment, housing, and transportation). Lastly, they use their influence to promote activities that support addressing social determinants "upstream," "midstream," and "downstream."

OMH also has a pilot initiative to redesign clinic services statewide as part of one of the eight identified SDMH-related activities, "regulation and licensing" (Rotter & Compton, 2020). This effort incorporates social determinant screening and support into the new regulations and includes stipulations addressing social determinants in program licensure. Another area of focus is educating the state workforce through various venues and platforms, including mandated modules on the State's learning management system, the OMH-supported Center for Practice Innovations (see below), conferences, statewide grand rounds, and community-based agency collaborations. OMH has expanded the level of training available to community-based providers on issues related to culture, equity, diversity, and inclusion by funding the addition of a Diversity Officer at the Center for Practice Innovations. This individual is responsible for creating, reviewing, and collaborating on training across the Center for Practice Innovations and helping providers statewide to better incorporate the National CLAS Standards. Also, to provide continuous, up-to-date information and strategies for reducing disparities in underrepresented populations, OMH hosts a bimonthly "Strategies for Behavioral Health Equity" webinar series. The webinar series has included topics such as "Practices/Approaches for Continuous Quality Improvement to Reduce Disparities for Marginalized Populations, Towards Inclusion & Anti-Oppression—The Challenge for Leadership", and "Racism: A Public Mental Health Crisis."

"Upstream and Midstream" Efforts at the Center for Practice Innovations

The New York State Office of Mental Health (OMH) and the Department of Psychiatry, Columbia University, established the Center for Practice Innovations (CPI) at Columbia Psychiatry and New York State Psychiatric Institute in 2007 to promote the widespread use of evidence-based practices developed for adults throughout New York State, so that it can effectively link the science (research and expertise of NYSPI/Columbia University) to real-world settings. CPI works with OMH to identify and involve clients, families, providers, agencies, communities, and scientific/academic organizations as partners in supporting the goals of OMH and the CPI.

The mission of the CPI is to help disseminate and implement evidence-based practices (EBPs) for people with behavioral health conditions and to educate and advance integrated care (CPI, 2023). As an intermediary organization, CPI bridges the gap between practice and research by supporting capacity building and sustaining EBPs within an agency or system. CPI's strong working relationship with OMH includes helping them think through policy, program guidance, licensing requirements, and the education of providers. The Center uses innovative approaches to build stakeholder collaborations, develop and maintain practitioners' expertise, and build agency infrastructures that support implementing and sustaining EBPs. CPI also supports community behavioral health providers to adapt to external factors that impact them, including training, strategies to remove barriers or work before starting the new practice, and supports for providers when implementing and sustaining an EBP.

CPI supports OMH's ongoing staff development by creating and disseminating synchronous and asynchronous training, technical assistance, and other educational opportunities. Training is available to OMH-licensed, Office of Addiction Services and Supports-certified (OASAS-certified), care managers, other not-for-profit behavioral health providers, and students working toward a degree to provide behavioral health care. The training supports the staff's professional development and the program's overall health, offering busy providers continuing education credits to NYS physicians, psychologists, nurses, licensed mental health counselors, licensed social workers, and substance misuse counselors. CPI provides continuing education credits for live in-person training, live webinars, self-study modules, and self-study archived webinars. CPI deploys synchronous and asynchronous training through a learning management system (LMS). The LMS allows service providers in various settings to access high-quality, evidence-based training/ best practices that help OMH and providers to offer:

▸ Culturally competent, person-centered care where recovery is possible and individualized for all service recipients

▸ Mental health services and support while reducing disparities in care and health status

▸ The promotion of mental and physical wellness, community inclusion, the translation of science to practice, and creating and sustaining a competent workforce

Through its various initiatives or practice competencies, CPI addresses cultural humility and SDH within training content. OMH and other licensing entities have mandated that Medicaid Managed Behavioral Health Network Providers companies within the State of New York must complete several required CPI training materials (i.e., "Cultural Competence", "Using the Cultural Formulation Interview", etc.) annually.

Systemic racism has pervasive impacts on those suffering from mental health conditions and those trying to alleviate that suffering. People from underrepresented communities, who are struggling, also grapple with discrimination, racism, stigma, and microaggressions, putting people from these communities at exceptionally high risk for adverse health and mental health outcomes. CPI works to develop and refine training that supports and expands the CLAS Standards by creating new racially, culturally, and structurally humble, justice-informed training for the frontline behavioral health workforce, including supervisors, care providers, peers, and advocates (i.e., "Foundations of the Social Determinants of Health", "Fundamentals of Antiracism for Behavioral Health Providers", etc.). This training content gives providers and trainees skills and tools, such as using social determinants and a culturally humble lens when working with individuals.

Conclusion

Equity in mental health, substance use, and physical health outcomes is achievable by addressing SDH through policy, programs, and environmental changes. Behavioral health organizations can also mitigate environmental stress and other health concerns through governance and leadership that promotes health equity through policy, practices, and allocated resources. More effective health care policies and practices would ensure that oversight organizations, service provider agencies, and communities intervene "upstream" by implementing social interventions to help prevent disabling and costly medical and mental disorders and improve public health. However, providers must also assess for and respond to the social determinants affecting people accessing care to address their financial, environmental, and social needs.

COLLEGE AND UNIVERSITY SCHOOL OF NURSING ADMINISTRATION

Nursing academia represents the starting point for all new nurses coming into the profession. The mission, vision, values, and philosophy of institutions flows through every nursing student, providing foundational influence on how each nurse practices. The policies and practices within schools of nursing addressing admissions, scholarship, attendance, and other factors must support the unique and sometimes, complex needs of potential and enrolled students. It is important that schools of nursing consider the Social Determinants of Learning (SDOL) alongside SSDH. These determinants are physical health, psychosocial health, physical environment, social environment, economic stability, and self-motivation. (Sanderson et al., 2021). Additionally, schools of nursing must recognize structural racism as being an underpinning cause of health disparities and develop strategies to address within its own structures and the classroom (Churchwell et al., 2020). Students entering nursing school must be greeted with not only a curriculum that addresses the structural racism as a root cause of health inequities but also inclusive policies to set the stage of expectations for practicing health equity as professional nurses. Considerations for policies and practices are offered below.

Student Recruitment and Developing Nursing Identity

Historically, gaining admission to nursing schools has been a highly competitive and challenging process (Santry, 2011; World, 2004). However, when examining applicant pools and the pipelines into nursing programs, it is crucial to consider the influence of SSDH. Several barriers hinder the recruitment of diverse students, including factors such as low economic status, inadequate prior education preparation, admission policies in higher education institutions, institutional bias, limited faculty diversity, and competition from other schools (Gates, 2018).

Prospective students from underrepresented backgrounds may be the first generation in their families to have the opportunity to attend college, and often require additional preparation and guidance to succeed. To address these barriers and promote diversity in nursing programs, outreach activities like university partnerships with middle and secondary schools are recommended. Engaging diverse faculty members in activities like visiting high school campus career fairs and offering campus tours is essential for reaching populations that may not otherwise consider a career in nursing. These partnerships can introduce students to nursing as a viable and accessible career option (Fontenut & McMurray, 2020).

Social and structural factors can impact the success of diverse students. These challenges include issues like imposter syndrome, inconsistent formal and institutional support, family support systems, peer pressure, the availability of emotional support, and racism (Bernard et al., 2020; Jackson et al., 2022; U.S. Department of Education, n.d.). One strategy for addressing these challenges and breaking down barriers related to identity, support, and role models is to involve university affinity groups in middle and secondary school outreach efforts. These groups can play a crucial role in providing guidance and support to prospective students, especially those who have been impacted by structural barriers in pursuing a nursing education. According to Musgrove et al. (2024) and Ali (2017), affinity groups foster a sense of belonging in education, establish community, and act as a foundation for institutional activism.

University, College, and School of Nursing Applicant Preparation and Qualifications

University admissions processes can be complex and may present barriers for potential nursing students, who may lack knowledge and guidance regarding the application and acceptance process (Wyness, 2017). Streamlining these processes is crucial to improving accessibility for such students. One effective strategy to simplify the pathway to nursing education is the implementation of Guided Pathways (California Community Colleges, 2024). This approach, as described by the California Community Colleges, aims to remove systemic obstacles by offering clear enrollment steps, course patterns, and support-centric support services. To make this strategy successful, it is essential to establish partnerships between secondary schools, community colleges, and universities, creating a seamless pipeline for aspiring nurses from various backgrounds to enter the profession.

Economic accessibility has gained prominence due to rising concerns about the levels of student loan debt. According to the Institute for Research on Poverty (2017) the cost of community college has risen by 70 percent, four-year public institutions by 160 percent, with Federal Pell grants covering only one third of tuition, compared to three fourths in 1980. Recent actions by the White House administration to alleviate this burden highlight the severity of the issue (Federal Student Aid, n.d.). To address these financial barriers, both states and higher educational institutions must take steps to enhance affordability. This can include offering more scholarship opportunities, ensuring manageable student loan costs, and offering grants to prospective students from diverse backgrounds. Both creative and traditional methods of securing funding for higher education should be explored in depth. Organizations such as college alumni and professional affinity groups may establish scholarships and grants to support historically excluded and underrepresented students. State and federal level grants should be secured to support students at the beginning of the educational journey, rather than to offset loans. Another consideration is to develop and strengthen dual enrollment programs, with class costs covered while the student is still in high school. Measures such as these and others are essential in tackling the economic domain of SSDH.

School of Nursing Admission Policies

Rethinking Standardized Tests

The use of standardized entrance exams as benchmarks for assessing adequate preparation for nursing school is a common practice. However, institutional policies related to testing methods and the use of test scores should be evaluated through a lens of diversity. According to the National Education Association (NEA) (Rosales & Walker, 2021), BIPOC (Black, Indigenous, and People of Color) students and students who are English language learners score lower on college entrance standardized exams than White students. It is recommended to assess traditional entry exams for any inherent bias. Some schools do not require standardized test scores for admission.

Holistic Admissions

In 2013, The American Association of Medical Colleges (AAMC) published an approach to health care admissions as a means to establish a comprehensive, flexible, and individualized approach to assessing a student's potential for success. This model is referred to as a Holistic Review. The core principles of Holistic Review are 1) broad-based selection criteria that align with the school's mission and goals; 2) evaluation of applicants based on a holistic perspective, considering their experiences, academic achievements, and personal attributes; and 3) assessment of an individual's contribution to the learning environment, with due weight given to all admission criteria (AAMC, 2024; Morrow, 2021; Witzburg & Sondheimer, 2013). These core principles reflect AAMC's updated language related to diversity and holistic admissions processes as of

September 2023, emphasizing three core values and removing the term "diversity." As of the time of writing, several state laws are being enacted that prohibit the use of terms like "diversity" and similar terms, often linking their use to the restriction of financial support (such as in the states of North Carolina, South Dakota, Tennessee, Oklahoma, Texas, Georgia, and Florida in 2023). This highlights the influence of politics on health outcomes and the ever-changing landscape of policies.

According to Fontenut and McMurray (2020), less than 50 percent of nursing schools employ a holistic process for selecting students, in contrast to 91% of medical schools and 93 percent of dentistry schools. Studies indicate that holistic admission practices are effective in enhancing diversity in the nursing workforce (Jung et al., 2021). Student outcomes using a holistic admission process reveal that graduation and licensure rates remain consistent with traditional metrics (Aul et al., 2022).

Considerations for implementing holistic admissions. Schools of nursing administrators, faculty, and staff must embody the ethical principles of the profession, which include addressing avoidable health inequalities throughout the School of Nursing. This process begins with a self-assessment of institutional missions and values to ensure alignment with SSDH considerations. With this, the organization can develop and apply a holistic lens. The logistical factors of implementation must include staff and faculty training in mitigating explicit and implicit bias. Participation in the review of applicants requires a lens of cultural humility combined with knowledge of the personal attributes such as integrity, leadership, honesty, innovation, intellectual curiosity, inclusive team player, and others considered necessary for success in health care professions and nursing (Harris et al., 2018).

The development or utilization of a rubric measuring readiness for nursing is necessary. This rubric should encompass measurements of critical thinking, teamwork, lived experiences, work ethic, educational and career goals, personal attributes, and potential contributions to the profession. Recommended interview methods include verbal, written, and simulation activities (Thompson & Sonke, 2021). These approaches, when combined with cognitive measurements, such as grade point average, provide an effective strategy for diversifying nursing student populations and, consequently, the nursing workforce.

Student Recruitment

The holistic admission process is one aspect of diversifying nursing student populations. In order to reach historically excluded and underrepresented individuals, proactive recruitment efforts must include outreach. One effective approach is to establish partnerships with K-12 schools and affinity nursing organizations. This step is essential to genuinely enhance and diversify the pool of applicants applying to any school of nursing. See Box 5.2 for an exemplar that illustrates this step.

Hiring: Diversification of Faculty

The Institute of Medicine (2003) has recommended enhancing the diversity of the nursing workforce as a means to address health disparities. Evidence indicates that increasing racial and ethnic diversity among non-nursing health care providers is associated with several benefits, including enhanced health care access, patient choice, and

BOX 5.2

Exemplar: Nursing Student Outreach Sponsored by Affinity Nursing Associations

The Capital City Black Nurses Association (2023) initiated an annual event, Breaking Down Barriers in Nursing, in partnership with the Sacramento Chapter of the Hispanic Nurses Association, The Hmong Nurses Association, and The Philippine Nurses Association for purpose of recruiting future BIPOC nursing students, known as Breaking Down Barriers to Nursing. Regional schools of nursing, including California State University, Sacramento, University of California, Davis, Betty Irene Moore School of Nursing, and several area community colleges are invited to attend this event, which has informational booths and faculty question-and-answer sessions. High school students are transported from the community at large to explore what it means to be a registered nurse, to discover pathways for acceptance to nursing school, and to learn about the mission, vision, and values of each organization.

satisfaction among historically excluded and underrepresented populations (Hoffman, 2016; Churchwell et al., 2020; Macias-Konstantopoulos et al., 2023). Additionally, it leads to better patient-provider communication and enriches the educational experiences of all health profession students (CDC, 2023).

Nurses who reflect and understand the unique needs of each patient in their care can provide more effective care, especially for patients from similar cultural backgrounds. This underscores the importance of having a diverse faculty to attract students from various cultures to pursue nursing careers. Moreover, the identification of structural and systemic racism is increasing, contributing to a deeper understanding of the relationship between racism and SSDH.

Social Justice Milieu

It is recommended that administrators regularly conduct evaluations of the social climate within each nursing program and throughout the departments at large. Social climate, in this context, refers to the perceptions held by members of a social group. It encompasses how individuals perceive their treatment, and the emotions they experience in response to personal and observed experiences within their defined group (Bennett, 2010). By conducting thorough and routine surveys, administrators can proactively identify concerning issues related to biased treatment, whether implicit or explicit. Areas deserving special attention include faculty-to-faculty interactions, faculty-to-student interactions, student-to-student interactions, staff-to-faculty interactions, and staff-to-student interactions. In clinically based programs, assessments of agency affiliates should also be incorporated into evaluations of the social climate. Considerations related to race, gender, religion, and age are critical areas for assessment to identify social and structural inequity and bias. According to Metzger et al. (2020) BIPOC students across all disciplines have reported experiencing racism, both subtle and direct, leading to feelings of being undervalued and alienated. Such experiences have led students from underrepresented groups to feel isolated and to seek out mentors of the same race. It is important to engage in strategies that can assist both

---

BOX 5.3

Exemplar: Educational Leadership: Addressing Racism in Nursing

The American Nurses Association—California (ANA/C) (2022) Taskforce to Eradicate Racism in Nursing has spearheaded efforts to understand the prevalence of racism in nursing clinical practice sites and schools of nursing in the State of California. Scholarly case study assessments for academic institutions are available, including the points of view of administrators, faculty, and students. The assessment allows for anonymous reporting, detailed feedback, and actionable suggested solutions for areas identified as needing improvement. Similar assessments are offered to health care institutions from the lens of both management and staff experiences.

---

students and faculty in fostering an accepting and positive social milieu that embraces diversity across all unique identifiers.

Integration of Implicit Bias Training Requirements

As of the time of writing, two states, California and Michigan, have implemented mandatory implicit bias training for nurses and other health care professionals. This development signifies a growing recognition and acceptance that bias plays a fundamental role in negative health outcomes, health disparities, and avoidable inequities. The incorporation of implicit bias training is beneficial when applied to both students and faculty. Organizations like the California Simulation Alliance (Health Impact, 2023) provide simulation activities designed for faculty and students to explore and address the role of implicit bias in health care. Further efforts across the nation should be adopted to make progress in recognizing and mitigating the impacts of implicit bias. See Box 5.3 for an exemplar that shows a strategy that one task force implemented to address racism in nursing.

IMPLICATIONS

Important policy priorities are to enhance provider, educator, and the emerging workforce awareness of the unrealized opportunities they have to improve health, reduce inequities, and develop policies that incentivize health care providers to be more proactive in the comprehensive provision of the care needed, so that every person has the fair opportunity to live their heathiest possible life. Effective interventions must be well designed and implemented; the more significant social and economic policies that impact the quality of life and the living conditions in homes and communities and the economic resources available to the household can also significantly affect health. Greater attention must be given to systematically evaluating social and economic policies that have health consequences. More importantly, policymakers, health care providers, and educators must use the currently available knowledge to improve the health of populations in their communities.

An SSDH framework and screening to capture social needs and to identify structural barriers can guide all levels of an organization to work toward a common purpose, with a common vocabulary, clear roles and responsibilities, and an agreed-upon goal. Platform integrations or integrating SDH screening tools can help organizations collect and interpret the data to drive intervention insights. Other partners, such as advisory boards, community partners, and community members, can also propel efforts forward and prove vital to the overall delivery of the intervention. Also, maximizing current spending by making supply chain or hiring decisions that considers SDH strategies, such as investing in local employment to help improve health outcomes.

CONCLUSION AND CALL TO ACTION

SSDH exert a significant influence and play a pivotal role in driving health inequities. Health care organizations and academic institutions hold a crucial responsibility in addressing SSDH and reducing health inequities. This role involves delivering high-quality health care and raising awareness about health inequities across all levels of their spheres of influence. To effectively address SSDH and contribute to the reduction of health inequities, health care systems, public health organizations, and academic institutions must develop policies and practices tailored to SSDH considerations. Recommendations are as follows:

> Advocate at institutional, community, city, state, and national levels. Utilization of the nursing voice is an essential component to address health inequity.
> Remove barriers to entering and advancing nursing professional practice.
> Develop partnerships supporting holistic needs of patients, including SSDH factors.
> Explore, examine, and address personal and institutional implicit bias.
> Create policies and care plans that center on understanding and integrating the context of SSDH factors in patient lives.
> Lead by example to encourage empathy, self-inquiry, discernment, and humility in others.

Challenging Thoughts to Consider

1. SSDH is a framework for discussion, targeted changes, progress, and evaluation while serving as a benchmark for everyone having the opportunity to live their healthiest possible life. What strategy can be used to determine whether an "impact has occurred, and the longevity of the action changed"?
2. What are strategies to advocate for policies that will remove barriers caused by structural determinants of health?
3. How might clinical practice and academic organizations partner with affinity nursing groups to better understand and meet the needs of historically excluded and underrepresented nurse populations?
4. What example can be identified that progress has occurred through "self-awareness of implicit bias"?
5. Discuss strategies that can be used to change the balance of power between patients and providers, evidenced by cultural humility.
6. Discuss self-reflection in transforming biases and attitudes toward diverse populations.

7. What strategies can schools of nursing use to gain the necessary administrative support and training to effectively implement holistic admission practices?

References

Alegría, M., NeMoyer, A., Falgàs Bagué, I., Wang, Y., & Alvarez, K. (2018). Social determinants of mental health: Where we are and where we need to go. *Current Psychiatry Reports, 20*(11), 95.

Ali, D. (2017). NASPA-Student Affairs Administrators in Higher Education. Safe spaces and brave spaces: Historical context and recommendations for student affairs professionals. *NASPA Policy and Practice Series*, Issue No. 2, 1–13.

American Association of Medical Colleges (AAMC). (2024). *Holistic admissions*. https://www.aamc.org/services/member-capacity-building/holistic-review

American Nurses Association. (n.d.). *Historical review*. https://www.nursingworld.org/~4ab5e0/globalassets/docs/ana/ana-expandedhistoricalreview.pdf

American Nurses Association–California. (2022). Assessments to eradicate racism in nursing. https://www.anacalifornia.org/racism-in-nursing-and-healthcare

Aul, K., Curry, K., & Johnson-Mallard, V. (2022). Outcomes of a holistic admissions process in a baccalaureate nursing program. *Teaching and Learning in Nursing, 17*(4), 350–356.

Banerjee, S., Paasche-Orlow, M. K., McCormick, D., Lin, M. Y., & Hanchate, A. D. (2021). Association between Medicare's hospital readmission reduction program and readmission rates across hospitals by Medicare bed share. *BMC Health Services Research, 21*(1), 248. https://doi.org/10.1186/s12913-021-06253-2

Batra, S., Orban, J., Zhang, H., Guterbock, T. M., Butler, L. A., Bogucki, C., & Chen, C. (2022). Analysis of social mission commitment at dental, medical, and nursing Schools in the US. *JAMA Network Open, 5*(5), e2210900. https://doi.org/10.1001/jamanetworkopen.2022.10900

Bay Area Regional Health Inequities Initiative (2015). Applying social determinants of health indicator data for advancing health equity. A guide for local health department epidemiologists and public health professions. Minnesota Department of Health.

Bennett, J. B. (2010). Social Climate Research. In I. B. Weiner, & W. E. Craighead (Eds.), *The corsini encyclopedia of psychology*. Wiley. https://doi.org/10.1002/9780470479216.corpsy0885

Bernard, D. L., Jones, S. C. T., & Volpe, V. V. (2020). Impostor phenomenon and psychological well-being: The moderating roles of John Henryism and school racial composition among black college students. *The Journal of Black Psychology, 46*(2–3), 195–227. https://doi.org/10.1177/0095798420924529

California Community Colleges. (2024). *Guided pathways*. https://www.cccco.edu/College-Professionals/Guided-Pathways

Capital City Black Nurses Association. (2023). *Breaking down barriers nursing conference*. https://www.ccbna.org/event-details/breaking-down-barriers-to-nursing-conference

Centers for Disease Control and Prevention. (2023). Gateway to health communication: Health equity guiding principles for inclusive communication. https://www.cdc.gov/healthcommunication/health_equity.html

Center for Practice Innovations at Columbia University. (2023). About. https://practiceinnovations.org/about

Churchwell, K., Elkind, M., Benjamin, R. M., Carson, A. P., Chang, E. K., Lawrence, W., Mills, A., Odom, T. M., Rodriguez, C. J., Rodriguez, F., Sanchez, E., Sharrief, A. Z., Sims, M., & Williams, O., On behalf of the American Heart Association. (2020). Call to action: Structural racism as a fundamental driver of health disparities: A Presidential advisory from the American Heart Association. *Circulation, 142*(24), e454–e468. https://doi.org/10.1161/CIR.0000000000000936

Cleveland, K. A., Motter, T., & Smith, Y., (2019). Affordable care: Harnessing the power of nurses. *OJIN: The Online Journal of Issues in Nursing, 24*(2).

Daniel-Robinson, L., & Moore, J. E. (2019). Innovation and opportunities to address social determinants of health in Medicaid managed care. *Institute for Medicaid Innovation*, pp. 1–24. https://healthystudent spromisingfutures.org/wp-content/uploads/2019/07/2019-IMI-Social_Determinants_of_Health_in_Medicaid-Report.pdf

de Mooij, L. D., Kikkert, M., Theunissen, J., Beekman, A. T. F., de Haan, L., Duurkoop, P. W. R. A., Van, H. L., & Dekker, J. J. M. (2019). Dying too soon: excess mortality in severe mental illness. *Frontiers in Psychiatry, 10*, 855. https://doi.org/10.3389/fpsyt.2019.00855

Doherty, J. A., Johnson, M., & McPheron, H. (2022). Advancing health equity through organizational change: Perspectives from heath care leaders. *Health Care Management Review, 47*(3), 263–270. https://doi.org/10.1097/HMR.0000000000000326

Federal Student Aid. (n.d.). The Biden-Harris Administration's student debt relief plan explained. https://studentaid.gov/debt-relief-announcement

Fontenut, J., & McMurray, P. (2020). Decolonizing entry to practice: Reconceptualizing methods to facilitate diversity in nursing programs. *Teaching & Learning in Nursing, 15*(4), 272–279. https://doi.org/10.1016/j.teln.2020.07.002

Fuller, L. L. (2016). Policy, advocacy, and activism: On bioethicists' role in combating racism. *American Journal of Bioethics, 16*(4), 29–31. https://doi.org/10.1080/15265161.2016.1145287

Fyfee, T. (2009). Nursing shaping and influencing health and social care policy. *Journal of Nursing Management, 17*, 698–706. https://doi.org/10.1111/j.1365-2834.2008.00946.x

Gates, S. A. (2018). What works in promoting and maintaining diversity in nursing programs. *Nursing Forum, 53*(2), 190–196. https://doi.org/10.1111/nuf.12242

Goulbourne, T., & Yanovitzky, I. (2021). The communication infrastructure as a social determinant of health: Implications for health policymaking and practice. *Milbank Q, 99*(1), 24–40. https://doi.org/10.1111/1468-0009.12496

Harris, T. B., Thomson, W. A., Moreno, N. P., Conrad, S., White, E., Young, G. H., Malmberg, E. D., Weisman, B., & Monroe, A. D. H. (2018). Advancing holistic review for faculty recruitment and advancement. *Academic Medicine, 93*(11), 1658–1662. https://comartsci.msu.edu/sites/default/files/documents/Advancing_Holistic_Review_for_Faculty_Recruit_Geraldine-Zeldes.pdf

Health Impact. (2023). California simulation alliance. https://healthimpact.org/programs/simulation/

Hoffman, K. M., Trawalter, S., Axt, J. R., & Oliver, M. N. (2016). Racial bias in pain assessment and treatment recommendations, and false beliefs about biological differences between blacks and whites. *Proceedings of the National Academy of Sciences of the United States of America, 113*(16), 4296–4301. https://doi.org/10.1073/pnas.1516047113

Institute for Research on Poverty. (2017). Financial barriers to college completion. University of Wisconsin-Madison. https://www.irp.wisc.edu/publications/factsheets/pdfs/FactSheet12-CollegeBarriers.pdf

Jackson, A., Colson-Fearon, B., & Versey, H. S. (2022). Managing intersectional invisibility and hypervisibility during the transition to college among first-generation women of color. *Psychology of Women Quarterly, 46*(3), 354–371. https://doi.org/10.1177/03616843221106087

Jackson, J. L., Grant, V., Barnett, K. S., Ball, M. K., Khalid, O., Texter, K., Laney, B., & Hoskinson, K. R. (2023). Structural racism, social determinants of health, and provider bias: Impact on brain development in critical congenital heart disease. *Canadian Journal of Cardiology, 39*(2), 133–143. https://doi.org/10.1016/j.cjca.2022.11.001

Jemal, A. (2017). Critical consciousness: a critique and critical analysis of the literature. *Urban Review, 49*(4), 602–626. https://doi.org/10.1007/s11256-017-0411-3

Jung, D., Latham, C., Fortes, K., & Schwartz, M. (2021). Using holistic admissions in pre-licensure programs to diversify the nursing workforce. *Journal of Professional Nursing, 37,* 359–365.

Kandasamy, V., Hirai, A. H., Kaufman, J. S., James, A. R., & Kotelchuck, M. (2020). Regional variation in Black infant mortality: The contribution of contextual factors. *PLoS One, 15*(8), e0237314. https://doi.org/10.1371/journal.pone.0237314

Lathrop, B. (2013). Nursing leadership in addressing the social determinants of health. *Policy, Politics, & Nursing Practice, 14*(1), 41–47. https://doi.org/10.1177/1527154413489887

Lee, J. P., Ponicki, W., Mair, C., Gruenewald, P., & Ghanem, L. (2020). What explains the concentration of off-premise alcohol outlets in Black neighborhoods? *SSM–Population Health, 12,* 100669.

Lewenson, S. (1996). *Taking charge: Nursing, suffrage & feminism in america 1873–1920.* National League for Nursing Press.

Macias-Konstantopoulos, W. L., Collins, K. A., Diaz, R., Duber, H. C., Edwards, C. D., Hsu, A. P., Ranney, M. L., Riviello, R. J., Wettstein, Z. S., & Sachs, C. J. (2023). Race, healthcare, and health disparities: a critical review and recommendations for advancing health equity. *Western Journal of Emergency Medicine, 24*(5), 906–918. https://doi.org/10.5811/westjem.58408

McKnight-Eily, L. R., Okoro, C. A., Strine, T. W., Verlenden, J., Hollis, N. D., Njai, R., Mitchell, E. W., Board, A., Puddy, R., & Thomas, C. (2021). Racial and ethnic disparities in the prevalence of stress and worry, mental health conditions, and increased substance use among adults during the COVID-19 pandemic–United States, April and May 2020. *MMWR. Morbidity and Mortality Weekly Report, 70*(5), 162–166.

Metzger, M., Dowling, T., Guinn, J., & Wilson, D. T. (2020). Inclusivity in baccalaureate nursing education: a scoping study. *Journal of Professional Nursing, 36*(1), 5–14. https://doi.org/10.1016/j.profnurs.2019.06.002

Momen, N. C., Plana-Ripoll, O., Agerbo, E., Christensen, M. K., Iburg, K. M., Laursen, T. M., Mortensen, P. B., Pedersen, C. B., Prior, A., Weye, N., & McGrath, J. J. (2022). Mortality associated with mental disorders and comorbid general medical conditions. *JAMA Psychiatry, 79*(5), 444–453.

Morrow, M. R. (2021). Holistic admission: What is it? How successful has it been in nursing, and what are the possibilities? *Nursing Science Quarterly, 34*(3), 256–262. https://doi.org/10.1177/08943184211010431

Musgrove, M. M. C., Ko, M. E., Schinske, J. N., & Corwin, L. A. (2024). Broadening participation in biology education research: a role for affinity groups in promoting social connectivity, self-efficacy, and belonging. *CBE—Life Sciences Education, 23*(1), ar8.

Nardi, D., Waite, R., Nowak, M., Hatcher, B., Hines-Martin, V., & Stacciarini, M. R. (2020). Achieving health equity through eradicating structural racism in the United States: A call to action for nursing leadership. *Journal of Nursing Scholarship, 52*(6), 696–704. https://doi.org/10.1111/jnu.12602

National Academy of Sciences, Engineering, and Medicine (NASEM), formerly the Institute of Medicine [IOM]. (2003). Health professions education: a bridge to quality. http://www.nap.edu/catalog/10681.html

National Academies of Sciences, Engineering, and Medicine (NASEM). (2021). *The future of nursing 2020–2030: charting a path to achieve health equity* (pp. 25982). National Academies Press. https://doi.org/10.17226/25982

National Academies of Sciences, Engineering, and Medicine (NASEM). (2019). *Criteria for selecting the leading health indicators for healthy people 2030. appendix e, healthy people 2030 framework.* National Academies Press. https://www.ncbi.nlm.nih.gov/books/NBK552645

National Institutes of Health. (2023). Societal benefits of improved health. Retrieved from https://www.nih.gov/about-nih/what-we-do/impact-nih-research/serving-society/societal-benefits-improved-health

National League for Nursing. (n.d.) History for the National League for Nursing, 1893–2018. https://www.nln.org/docs/default-source/uploadedfiles/default-document-library/nln-timeline-june-2020.pdf?sfvrsn=16f6a70d_0

National League for Nursing (NLN). (2021). Taking aim: Addressing racism, diversity, equity, inclusion, bias, and social justice. https://www.nlntakingaimdei.org/

National League for Nursing (NLN). (2024). Public Policy. https://www.nln.org/public-policy

National Leage for Nursing/Walden University Institute for Social Determinants of Health and Social Change. (n.d.). https://www.nlnwaldensdoh.org/

NIDA. (2022, September 27). Part 1: The connection between substance use disorders and mental illness. https://nida.nih.gov/publications/research-reports/common-comorbidities-substance-use-disorders/part-1-connection-between-substance-use-disorders-mental-illness

Office of Disease Prevention and Health Promotion. (n.d.). Healthy People 2030. U.S. Department of Health and Human Services. https://health.gov/healthypeople

Office of Health Promotion and Illness Prevention. (2022). Health equity and health disparities and environmental scan. https://health.gov/sites/default/files/2022-04/HP2030-HealthEquityEnvironmentalScan.pdf

Office of Mental Health (OMH). (n.d.). About Us. https://omh.ny.gov/omhweb/about/

Patient Protection and Affordable Care Act H.R. 3590 (2010). https://www.congress.gov/bill/111th-congress/house-bill/3590

Pevalin, D. J., Reeves, A., Baker, E., & Bentley, R. (2017). The impact of persistent poor housing conditions on mental health: a longitudinal population-based study. *Preventive Medicine*, *105*, 304–310.

Rambachan, A., Abe-Jones, Y., Fernandez, A., & Shahram, Y. (2022). Racial disparities in 7-Day readmissions from an adult hospital medicine service. *Journal of Racial and Ethnic Health Disparities*, *9*(4), 1500–1505. https://doi.org/10.1007/s40615-021-01088-3

Ribisl, K. M., D'Angelo, H., Feld, A. L., Schleicher, N. C., Golden, S. D., Luke, D. A., & Henriksen, L. (2017). Disparities in tobacco marketing and product availability at the point of sale: Results of a national study.

Preventive Medicine, *105*, 381–388. https://doi.org/10.1016/j.ypmed.2017.04.010

Roper, W. L., Baker, E. L., Dyal, W. W., & Nicola, R. M. (1992). Strengthening the public health system. *Public Health Reports*. *107*(6), 609–615.

Rosales, J., & Walker, T. (2021). The racist beginnings of standardized testing. *NEA Today*. https://www.nea.org/nea-today/all-news-articles/racist-beginnings-standardized-testing

Rotter, M., & Compton, M. T. (2020). The social determinants of mental health: A white paper detailing promising practices and opportunities at the New York State office of mental health. https://omh.ny.gov/omhweb/sdmh-white-paper.pdf

Sanderson, C. D., Hollinger-Smith, L. M., & Cox, K. (2021). Developing a social determinants of health learning framework: A case study. *Nurse Education Perspectives*, *42*, 205–211.

Santry, C. (2011). Students face stiff competition. *Nursing Times*, *107*(1), 3.

Shim, R. S., & Compton, M. T. (2018). Addressing the social determinants of mental health: If not now, when? If not us, who? *Psychiatric Services (Washington, D.C.)*, *69*(8), 844–846.

Singh, G. K., & Yu, S. M. (2019). Infant mortality in the United States, 1915–2017: large social inequalities have persisted for over a century. *International Journal of MCH and AIDS*, *8*(1), 19–31. https://doi.org/10.21106/ijma.271

Solar, O., & Irwin, A. (2010). *A conceptual framework for action on the social determinants of health*. World Health Organization.

Thompson, T., & Sonke, A. (2021). Multiple mini interviews as part of holistic admissions review for nursing schools. *Journal of Professional Nursing*, *37*(6), 1086–1091. https://doi.org/10.1016/j.profnurs.2021.08.009

U.S. Department of Education. (n.d.). Supporting child and student social, emotional, behavioral and mental health needs. https://www2.ed.gov/documents/students/supporting-child-student-social-emotional-behavioral-mental-health.pdf

U.S. Department of Health and Human Services (USDHHS). Office of Health Promotion and Illness Prevention. (2022). About ODPHP. https://health.gov/about-odphp

U.S. Department of Health and Human Services, Office of Minority Health. (n.d). https://minorityhealth.hhs.gov/

U.S. Department of Health and Human Service. Office of Minority Health. (2022). Infant mortality and African Americans. https://minorityhealth.hhs.gov/omh/browse.aspx?lvl=4&lvlid=23

U.S. Department of Health and Human Services, Office of Minority Health. (2022). Infant mortality and Black Americans. What is infant mortality? https://minorityhealth.hhs.gov/infant-mortality-and-african-americans

U.S. Department of Health and Human Services, Office of Minority Health. (2016). National standards for culturally and linguistically appropriate services in health and health care: Compendium of state-sponsored national CLAS standards implementation activities. https://thinkculturalhealth.hhs.gov/clas

Witzburg, R. A., & Sondheimer, H. M. (2013). Holistic Review—Shaping the medical profession one applicant at a time. *New England Journal of Medicine*, *368*(17), 1565–1567.

World, H. (2004). Whatever it takes. *NurseWeek California*, *17*(25), 33.

Wyness, G. (2017). Rules of the game: disadvantaged students and the university admission process. *The Sutton Trust*. https://www.suttontrust.com/our-research/rules-of-the-game-university-admissions/

Zappas, M., Walton-Moss, B., Sanchez, C., Hildebrand, J. A., & Kirkland, T. (2021). The decolonization of nursing education. *Journal for Nurse Practitioners*, *17*(2), 225–29. https://doi.org/10.1016/j.nurpra.2020.11.006